Ninja Air Fryer Cookbook

for Beginners

100+ Quick, Easy and Delicious Recipes for the Ninja Air Fryer and Max XL (Beginners and Advanced Users)

Table of Contents

Introduction

Are you looking for a meal plan full of flavorsome, crispy, and oil-free delights? Then you have landed at the right place! This cookbook brings you all eighty delicious recipes that are fried, roasted, or dehydrated in the Ninja Foodi Air Fryer!

A healthy diet and effortless cooking, that's the kind of combination that we all look for. But our cringe for crispy snacks and fast food makes it impossible to enjoy fat-free, low caloric meals. But not anymore! Today if you have an Air Fryer as good as the Ninja Foodi AF101, you can cook all sorts of meals with 70 percent fewer fats. The powerful Ninja Foodi Air Fryer comes with 4 cooking operations so that you could cook a variety of meals in a different style in a single pot. With this Air Fryer, you can: Air Fry, Roast, and Dehydrate your food any time. The user-friendly control panel lets you use all the cooking operations using the presets or the manual settings. The cooking time and temperature can be easily adjusted to cook veggies, fruits, bread, beef, lamb, pork, steaks, poultry, and even dessert,

These 4 one multipurpose kitchen companions come with a 4-quart food holding capacity, which is great to cook food for an average size family. All the accessories, including the Air Fryer basket and its crisper plate, are ceramic coated, which make cleaning easy. And with the Reheat option, you can easily heat leftover crispy snacks and food without making it lose the texture. Perhaps, there is a list of perks that goes on when it comes to the Ninja Food Air Fryer. And if you are ready to get the best of this kitchen appliance, then scroll more and find out a whole range of recipes created and cooked using the Ninja Foodi Air Fryer. These luscious recipes are simple enough to try on the routine base and tasty enough to serve all your special guests and loved ones. In this Ninja Foodi Air Fryer cookbook, you will get to learn how to cook oil-free snacks, breakfast, desserts, turkey, chicken, steaks, and pork chops in just a few minutes. So, let's get started!

Chapter 1: Breakfast Recipes

1. Cheesy Sausage Casserole

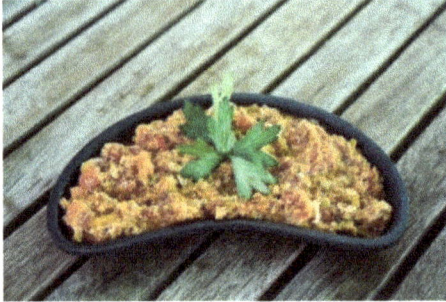

Prep Time: 15 minutes.

Cook Time: 15 minutes.

Serves: 8

Ingredients:

- 1 tablespoon olive oil
- 1 lb ground sausage
- 1/4 cup white onion, diced
- 1 red bell pepper, diced
- 8 eggs, beaten
- 1/2 cup Colby jack cheese, shredded
- 1 teaspoon fennel seed
- 1/2 teaspoon garlic salt

Preparation:

1. Sauté onion, sausage, and bell pepper in a cooking pan with olive oil for 5-7 minutes. until veggies are soft.
2. Transfer this mixture to a 6 inches baking pan.
3. Crack whole eggs in a glass bowl, and beat them with a fork.
4. Stir in fennel seed and garlic salt. Mix and pour into the pan.
5. Drizzle cheese on top and place this pan in the Air Fryer basket.
6. Return the Air Fryer basket to the Air Fryer.
7. Select the Air Fry mode at 390 degrees F for 15 minutes.
8. Once done, remove the basket and the pan from the Air Fryer.
9. Scramble and serve warm.

Serving Suggestion: Serve the casserole with toasted bread slices.

Variation Tip: Ground chicken or beef can also be used instead of ground sausage.

Nutritional Information Per Serving:

Calories 305 | Fat 25g |Sodium 532mg | Carbs 2.3g | Fiber 0.4g | Sugar 2g | Protein 18.3g

2. Scrambled Eggs

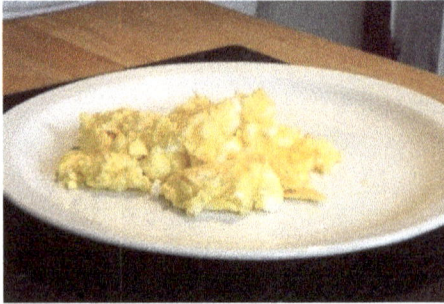

Prep Time: 10 minutes.

Cook Time: 20 minutes.

Serves: 6

Ingredients:

- 4 tablespoon butter, melted
- 6 eggs, beaten
- Salt and black pepper, to taste
- 2/3 cup heavy cream
- 1 cups mozzarella cheese, shredded

Preparation:

1. Beat eggs with salt, black pepper, cream, and butter in a bowl.
2. Pour the mixture into a greased 6 inches baking pan and drizzle cheese on top.
3. Place the prepared pan in the Air Fryer basket.
4. Return the Air Fryer basket to the Air Fryer.
5. Select the Air Fry mode at 350 degrees F for 10 minutes.
6. Stir the egg mixture with a fork, then return to the Air Fryer again.
7. Cook another 10 minutes. at 350 degrees F on Air Fryer mode.
8. Serve.

Serving Suggestion: Serve the eggs with toasted bread slices and crispy bacon.

Variation Tip: Add herbed cream to the eggs.

Nutritional Information Per Serving:

Calories 190 | Fat 18g |Sodium 150mg | Carbs 0.6g | Fiber 0.4g | Sugar 0.4g | Protein 7.2g

3. Banana Bread

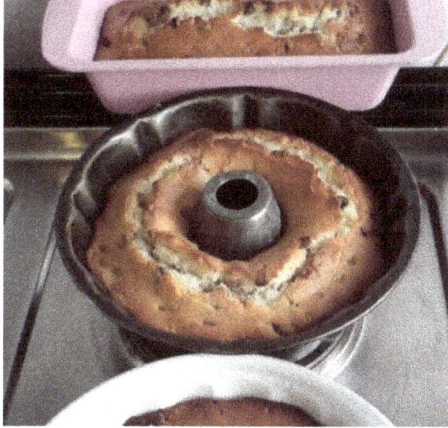

Prep Time: 10 minutes.
Cook Time: 28 minutes.
Serves: 6

Ingredients:

- 3/4 cup all-purpose flour
- 1/4 teaspoon baking soda
- 1/4 teaspoon salt
- 1 egg
- 2 bananas overripe, mashed
- 1/2 teaspoon vanilla
- 1/4 cup sour cream
- 1/4 cup vegetable oil
- 1/2 cup sugar

Preparation:

1. Mash bananas in a suitable bowl and add vanilla, sour cream, vegetable oil, and egg.
2. Beat these ingredients until well incorporated.
3. Stir in all-purpose flour, sugar, baking soda, and salt.
4. Mix well to get a smooth and thick batter.
5. Pour this batter into a greased 7 inches Bundt pan.
6. Place this Bundt pan in the Air Fryer basket
7. Return the Air Fryer basket to the Air Fryer.
8. Select the Air Fry mode at 310 degrees F for 28 minutes.
9. Once done, remove the basket and the pan from the Air Fryer.
10. Transfer the cake to a wire rack and allow it to cool.
11. Slice and serve.

Serving Suggestion: Serve the bread slices with cream cheese spread.

Variation Tip: Add raisins to the batter.

Nutritional Information Per Serving:

Calories 267 | Fat 12g |Sodium 165mg | Carbs 39g | Fiber 1.4g | Sugar 22g | Protein 3.3g

4. Vegetable Frittata

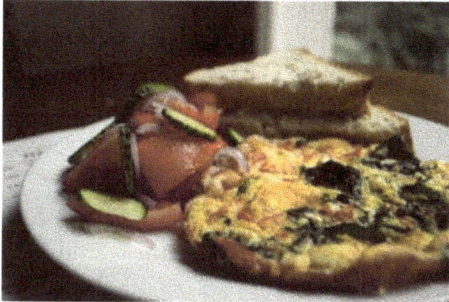

Prep Time: 15 minutes.

Cook Time: 27 minutes.

Serves:6

Ingredients:

- 2 teaspoons olive oil
- 6 ounces sausage Links
- ¼ cup red bell pepper, chopped
- ¼ cup yellow onion, chopped
- 5 eggs
- ¼ teaspoon kosher salt
- ¼ teaspoon ground black pepper
- ½ cup kale leaves, chopped
- 1-ounce goat cheese, crumbled

Preparation:

1. Sauté sausage links with 2 teaspoons of olive oil in a skillet for 4 minutes.
2. Stir in onions and peppers, then cook for 3 minutes. until soft.
3. Grease an 8 inches grease pan and spread the sausage mixture in it.
4. Whisk eggs with kale, black pepper, and salt in a bowl.
5. Pour this mixture over the pepper mixture and place the pan in the Air Fryer basket.
6. Return the Air Fryer basket to the Air Fryer.
7. Select the Air Fry mode at 330 degrees F for 10 minutes.
8. Slice and serve.

Serving Suggestion: Serve the frittata with toasted bread slices and crispy bacon.

Variation Tip: Broil the frittata with mozzarella cheese on top.

Nutritional Information Per Serving:

Calories 183 | Fat 15g | Sodium 402mg | Carbs 2.5g | Fiber 0.4g | Sugar 1.1g | Protein 10g

5. Tomato Frittata

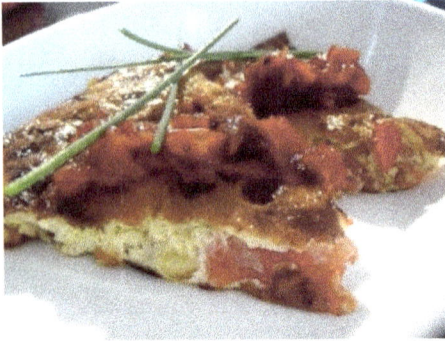

Prep Time: 10 minutes.

Cook Time: 6 minutes.

Serves: 4

Ingredients:

- 4 eggs
- 3 tablespoons heavy cream
- 2 bacon slices, cooked and crumbled
- ½ cup Jack cheese, shredded
- ¼ cup green chiles, chopped
- 3 tablespoons tomatoes, diced
- 2 tablespoons onion, chopped
- Salt and ground black pepper, to taste

Preparation:

1. At 350 degrees F, preheat your Ninja Air Fryer on Air Fry mode.
2. Grease a 6 inches pan with cooking spray.
3. Beat eggs with cream, bacon, cheese, black pepper, salt, onion, tomatoes, and chiles in a bowl.
4. Pour this mixture into the pan and set this pan in the Air Fryer basket.
5. Return the Air Fryer basket to the Air Fryer and cook for 6 minutes.
6. Garnish as desired.
7. Slice and serve warm.

Serving Suggestion: Serve the frittata with sautéed tomatoes or sausages on top.

Variation Tip: Add chopped bell peppers to the frittata.

Nutritional Information Per Serving:

Calories 273 | Fat 22g |Sodium 517mg | Carbs 3.3g | Fiber 0.2g | Sugar 1.4g | Protein 16.1g

6. Egg Bites

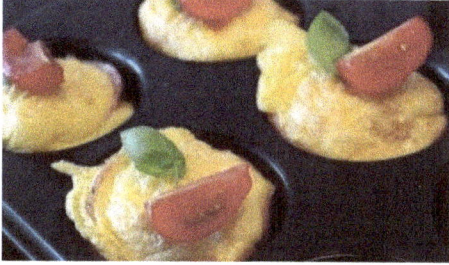

Prep Time: 10 minutes.
Cook Time: 10 minutes.
Serves: 6

Ingredients:

- 5 eggs
- 1/4 cup heavy whipping cream
- 1 teaspoon salt
- 1/2 teaspoon pepper
- 1/4 cup ham, diced
- 1/4 cup mushrooms, chopped
- 1/4 cup tomatoes, diced
- 1/4 cup green onions, chopped
- 1/4 cup cheddar cheese, shredded

Preparation:

1. Beat eggs with black pepper, salt, and cream in a suitable mixing bowl.
2. Stir in ham, mushrooms, tomatoes, green onions, and mix gently.
3. Divide the mixture into a suitable muffin mold.
4. Place the mold in the Air Fryer basket.
5. Return the Air Fryer basket to the Air Fryer.
6. Select the Air Fry mode at 310 degrees F for 10 minutes.
7. Once done, remove the basket and the pan from the Air Fryer.
8. Serve.

Serving Suggestion: Serve the eggs bites with fresh vegetable garnishing.

Variation Tip: Add dried herbs to the egg batter.

Nutritional Information Per Serving:
Calories 102 | Fat 7.6g |Sodium 545mg | Carbs 1.5g | Fiber 0.4g | Sugar 0.7g | Protein 7.1g

7. Breakfast Pizza

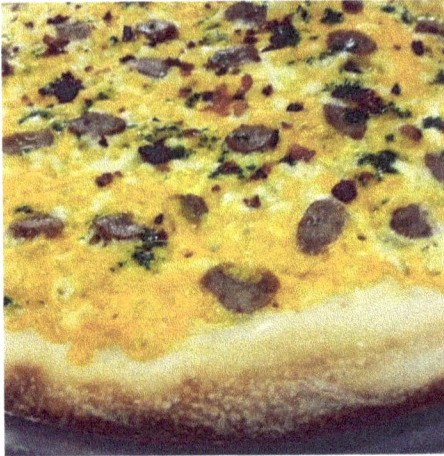

Prep Time: 15 minutes.
Cook Time: 16 minutes.
Serves: 6

Ingredients:

Pizza dough

- 1 cup all-purpose flour
- 1 tablespoon granulated sugar
- 1 teaspoon baking powder
- 1/4 teaspoon kosher salt
- 2/3 cup Greek yogurt

Toppings

- 4 bacon slices, cut into thin strips
- 4 eggs, beaten
- 2 oz cream cheese, softened
- 2 oz cheese, shredded

Preparation:

1. Add flour, baking powder, salt, and sugar in a mixing bowl, then mix well.
2. Stir in yogurt and mix to get a crumbly mixture.
3. Transfer the dough to a working surface and knead well.
4. Spread the dough into a circle 8 inch in diameter.
5. Line the Air Fryer basket with parchment paper and place the crust in it.
6. Brush the crust with milk, egg whites, and butter.
7. Return the Air Fryer basket to the Air Fryer.
8. Select the Air Fry mode at 375 degrees F for 10 minutes.
9. Once done, remove the basket and the pan from the Air Fryer.

10. Flip the crust and continue Air Frying for 3 minutes.
11. Meanwhile, sauté bacon in a skillet until brown.
12. Stir in eggs and cook until it makes a scramble.
13. Top the pizza crust with egg mixture and cheese.
14. Air Fry for another 3 minutes. in the Air Fryer.
15. Serve warm.

Serving Suggestion: Serve the pizza with your hot sauce or cheese dip.

Variation Tip: Use crispy pepperoni slices to top pizza.

Nutritional Information Per Serving:

Calories 282 | Fat 15g |Sodium 526mg | Carbs 20g | Fiber 0.6g | Sugar 3.3g | Protein 16g

8. Zucchini Frittata

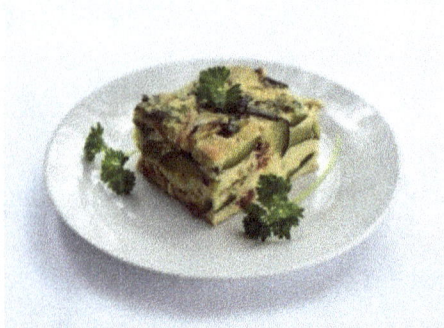

Prep Time: 10 minutes.
Cook Time: 28 minutes.
Serves: 4

Ingredients:

- 1 tablespoon butter
- 1 onion, sliced
- 1 large zucchini, sliced
- ½ teaspoon of sea salt
- ¼ teaspoon ground black pepper
- 3 eggs
- ½ cup heavy cream
- ¼ teaspoon ground nutmeg
- 1 cup Gouda cheese, shredded

Preparation:

1. At 425 degrees F, preheat your Ninja Air Fryer on Air Fry mode.
2. Sauté onion with butter in a skillet for 5 minutes.
3. Stir in zucchini and sauté for 3 minutes.
4. Season with salt and black pepper, then transfer to a bowl.
5. Add cream, nutmeg and eggs, then beat the mixture.
6. Pour this mixture into a 7 inches pan and place this pan in the Air Fryer basket.
7. Return the Air Fryer basket to the Air Fryer.
8. Select the Air Fry mode at 425 degrees F for 20 minutes.
9. Slice and serve warm.

Serving Suggestion: Serve the frittata with toasted bread slices and crispy bacon.

Variation Tip: Add sliced bell peppers to the frittata.

Nutritional Information Per Serving:
Calories 237 | Fat 19g |Sodium 518mg | Carbs 7g | Fiber 1.5g | Sugar 3.4g | Protein 12g

9. Breakfast Potatoes

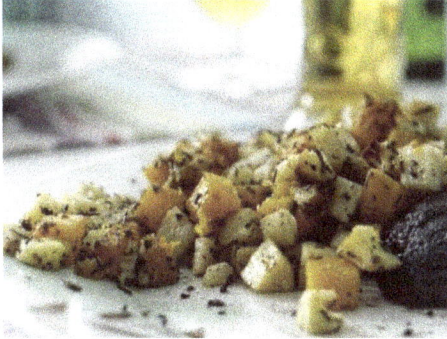

Prep Time: 15 minutes.
Cook Time: 35 minutes.
Serves: 4

Ingredients:

- 1 1/2 lbs baby potatoes, diced
- 1 large red bell pepper, diced
- 1 large green bell pepper, diced
- 2 tablespoons olive oil
- 2 teaspoons garlic powder
- 1 teaspoon onion powder
- 1 teaspoon black pepper
- 1/2 teaspoon kosher salt
- 1 teaspoon dried herbs

Preparation:

1. Toss potatoes with peppers, olive oil, dried herbs, onion powder, black pepper, salt, and garlic in a large bowl.
2. Spread the potatoes and peppers in an Air Fryer basket.
3. Return the Air Fryer basket to the Air Fryer.
4. Select the Air Fry mode at 400 degrees F for 35 minutes.
5. Toss the potatoes after every 10 minutes. and resume cooking.
6. Serve warm.

Serving Suggestion: Serve the potatoes with crispy bacon or sautéed green beans.

Variation Tip: Add diced sweet potatoes and yellow squash to the mixture.

Nutritional Information Per Serving:
Calories 209 | Fat 7.5g |Sodium 321mg | Carbs 34.1g | Fiber 4g | Sugar 3.8g | Protein 4.3g

10. Breakfast Croquettes

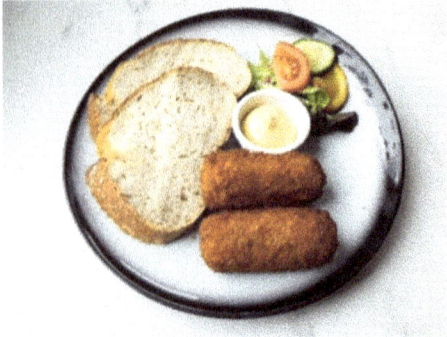

Prep Time: 15 minutes.
Cook Time: 14 minutes.
Serves: 12

Ingredients:

- 3 tablespoons butter
- 3 tablespoons all-purpose flour
- 3/4 cup milk
- 6 hard-boiled eggs, chopped
- 1/2 cup fresh asparagus, chopped
- 1/2 cup green onions, chopped
- 1/3 cup cheddar cheese, shredded
- 1 tablespoon fresh tarragon, minced
- 1/4 teaspoon salt
- 1/4 teaspoon black pepper
- 1 ¾ cups panko bread crumbs
- 3 eggs, beaten
- Cooking spray

Preparation:

1. Set a suitable saucepan over medium heat, and add butter to melt.
2. Slowly stir in flour and cook for 2 minutes. with continuous stirring.
3. Add milk, mix and cook until the mixture thickens.
4. Add eggs, green onions, asparagus, tarragon, salt, black pepper, and cheese.
5. Mix and cook for 2 minutes. until the cheese is melted. Allow the filling to cool.
6. At 350 degrees F, preheat the Air Fryer on Air Fryer mode.
7. Make 12 - 3 inches ball out of this mixture.
8. Beat 3 eggs in one bowl and spread breadcrumbs in a plate.
9. Dip the balls in the eggs and coat them with breadcrumbs.
10. Place the balls in the Air Fryer basket and spray them with cooking oil.
11. Return the Air Fryer basket to the Air Fryer.

12. Select the Air Fry mode at 350 degrees F for 10 minutes.
13. Once done, remove the basket and the pan from the Air Fryer.
14. Serve warm.

Serving Suggestion: Serve the croquettes with a garlic mayo dip and fresh bread.

Variation Tip: Use crushed cornflakes for breading to have extra crisp.

Nutritional Information Per Serving:

Calories 199 | Fat 11.1g |Sodium 297mg | Carbs 14.9g | Fiber 1g | Sugar 2.5g | Protein 9.9g

Chapter 2: Snacks and Appetizers

1. Pepperoni Chips

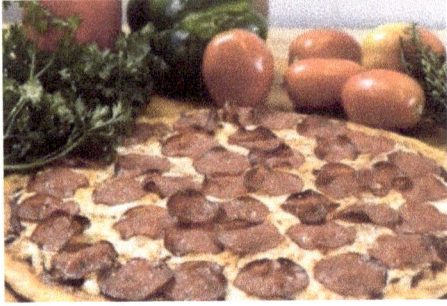

Prep Time: 10 minutes.
Cook Time: 8 minutes.
Serves: 5

Ingredients:

- 10 pepperoni slices

Preparation:

1. Spread the pepperoni in the Air Fryer basket in a single layer.
2. Return the Air Fryer basket to the Air Fryer.
3. Select the Air Fry mode at 360 degrees F for 8 minutes.
4. Toss and flip the fries in the basket once cooked halfway through.
5. Return the basket and resume the cooking.
6. Serve warm.

Serving Suggestion: Serve with tomato sauce or on top of the pizza.

Variation Tip: Dehydrate the slices for crisper.

Nutritional Information Per Serving:
Calories 100 | Fat 2g |Sodium 480mg | Carbs 4g | Fiber 2g | Sugar 0g | Protein 18g

2. Zucchini Chips

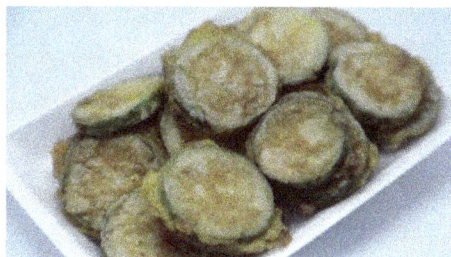

Prep Time: 15 minutes.
Cook Time: 12 minutes.
Serves: 2

Ingredients:

- 1 medium zucchini, cut into chips
- 1 egg, beaten
- 3/4 cup panko crumbs
- 1/4 cup parmesan cheese
- Olive oil spray

Preparation:

1. Mix parmesan cheese and breadcrumbs in a mixing bowl.
2. Whisk and beat the egg in a bowl.
3. Dip the zucchini in the egg and then coat with breadcrumbs.
4. Spread the coated zucchini slices in the Air Fryer basket.
5. Return the Air Fryer basket to the Air Fryer.
6. Select the Air Fry mode at 400 degrees F for 12 minutes.
7. Flip the zucchini chips once cooked halfway through.
8. Serve warm.

Serving Suggestion: Serve with mayonnaise or cream cheese dip.

Variation Tip: Use crushed cornflakes for breading to have extra crisp.

Nutritional Information Per Serving:
Calories 180 | Fat 3.2g |Sodium 133mg | Carbs 32g | Fiber 1.1g | Sugar 1.8g | Protein 9g

3. Jalapeno Poppers

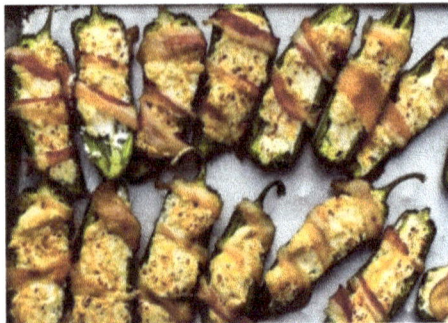Prep Time: 10 minutes.

Cook Time: 8 minutes.

Serves: 10

Ingredients:

- 10 jalapenos, cut in half lengthwise
- 10 bacon slices
- 8 oz cream cheese, room temperature
- 1 teaspoon cumin
- 1 cup Monterey jack cheese, shredded
- Olive oil spray

Preparation:

1. Whisk cream cheese, cheese, and cumin in a mixing bowl.
2. Divide this mixture into the jalapeno's halves.
3. Wrap the stuffed jalapeno with one bacon slices and secure with a toothpick.
4. Place the stuffed and wrapped jalapenos in the Air Fryer basket.
5. Return the Air Fryer basket to the Air Fryer.
6. Select the Air Fry mode at 370 degrees F for 8 minutes.
7. Serve warm.

Serving Suggestion: Serve with tomato sauce or cream cheese dip.

Variation Tip: Stuff the filling in bell pepper cups, then Air Fry with crispy bacon on top.

Nutritional Information Per Serving:

Calories 229 | Fat 1.9 |Sodium 567mg | Carbs 1.9g | Fiber 0.4g | Sugar 0.6g | Protein 11.8g

4. Fried Artichoke Hearts

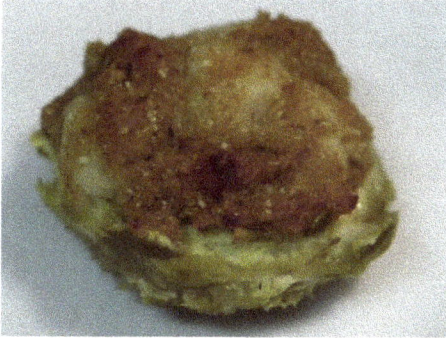

Prep Time: 10 minutes.
Cook Time: 15 minutes.
Serves: 4

Ingredients:

- 3 cans quartered artichokes, drained
- 1/2 cup mayonnaise
- 1 cup panko breadcrumbs
- ⅓ cup parmesan, grated
- Salt and black pepper, to taste
- Sprinkle of parsley for garnish

Preparation:

1. Place the artichokes in a colander and let them drain.
2. Pat them dry and transfer to a plate.
3. Mix mayonnaise, black pepper, and salt in a small bowl.
4. Stir in artichokes and mix well to coat.
5. Dredge the artichokes through the breadcrumbs to coat.
6. Place the coated artichokes in the Air Fryer basket.
7. Return the Air Fryer basket to the Air Fryer.
8. Select the Air Fry mode at 370 degrees F for 15 minutes.
9. Drizzle parmesan cheese on top and serve.

Serving Suggestion: Serve with mayonnaise or cream cheese dip.

Variation Tip: Use crushed cornflakes for breading to have extra crisp.

Nutritional Information Per Serving:
Calories 185 | Fat 11g |Sodium 355mg | Carbs 21g | Fiber 5.8g | Sugar 3g | Protein 4.7g

5. Buffalo Cauliflower

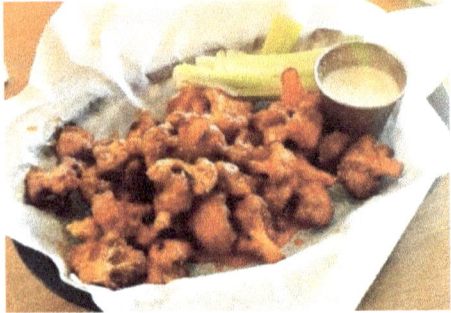

Prep Time: 15 minutes.
Cook Time: 20 minutes.
Serves: 4

Ingredients:

- 2 cups cauliflower florets
- Olive oil spray
- ½ cup hot sauce
- ¾ cup nutritional yeast

Preparation:

1. At 400 degrees F, preheat your Ninja Air Fryer on Air Fry mode.
2. Spread the cauliflower in a suitable tray and spray them with cooking oil.
3. Drizzle hot sauce and yeast on top, then toss well.
4. Transfer the cauliflower to the Air Fryer basket.
5. Return the Air Fryer basket to the Air Fryer and cook for 20 minutes.
6. Toss the cauliflower after every 5 minutes.
7. Serve warm.

Serving Suggestion: Serve with mayonnaise dip and celery sticks.

Variation Tip: Use BBQ sauce to season the cauliflower florets.

Nutritional Information Per Serving:
Calories 122 | Fat 1.8g |Sodium 794mg | Carbs 17g | Fiber 8.9g | Sugar 1.6g | Protein 14.9g

6. Fried Pickles

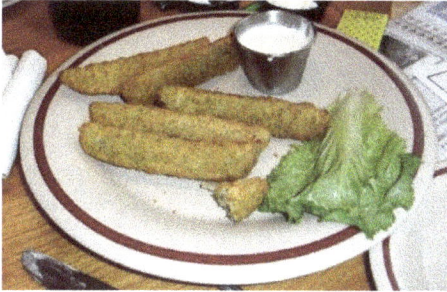

Prep Time: 10 minutes.

Cook Time: 7 minutes.

Serves: 12

Ingredients:

- 12 pickles spears
- 1 cup coconut flour
- 2 ½ oz pork rinds
- 2 eggs

Preparation:

1. Cut the pickles into a spear and pat them dry.
2. Beat eggs in one bowl and spread coconut flour.
3. Crush the pork rinds in a food processor and transfer to a bowl.
4. First coat the pickle spears in the flour, then dip in the egg and finally cover with pork rinds.
5. Place the coated pickle in the Air Fryer basket.
6. Return the Air Fryer basket to the Air Fryer.
7. Select the Air Fry mode at 400 degrees F for 7 minutes.
8. Flip the chips once cooked halfway through.
9. Serve warm.

Serving Suggestion: Serve with mayonnaise or cream cheese dip.

Variation Tip: Use crushed cornflakes for breading to have extra crisp.

Nutritional Information Per Serving:

Calories 163 | Fat 11.5g |Sodium 918mg | Carbs 8.3g | Fiber 4.2g | Sugar 0.2g | Protein 7.4g

7. Fried Shrimp

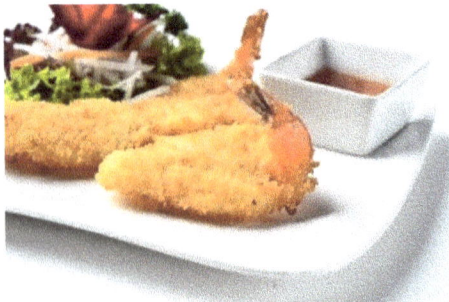

Prep Time: 15 minutes.

Cook Time: 6 minutes.

Serves: 10

Ingredients:

- 1 cup Italian bread crumbs
- 1 tablespoon taco seasoning
- 1 tablespoon garlic salt
- 4 tablespoons butter, melted
- 17-20 shrimp, shells removed, deveined
- Olive oil spray

Preparation:

1. Mix breadcrumbs with seasonings in a mixing bowl.
2. At 400 degrees F, preheat your Ninja Air Fryer on Air Fry mode.
3. Add butter to a suitable bowl and heat it for 30 seconds to melt in the microwave.
4. Dip the shrimp in the melted butter, then coat with breadcrumbs.
5. Place the coated shrimp in the Air Fryer basket.
6. Return the Air Fryer basket to the Air Fryer.
7. Select the Air Fry mode at 400 degrees F for 5 minutes.
8. Flip the shrimp once cooked halfway through.
9. Serve warm.

Serving Suggestion: Serve with tomato or sweet chili sauce.

Variation Tip: Use crushed cornflakes for breading to have extra crisp.

Nutritional Information Per Serving:

Calories 134 | Fat 5.9g |Sodium 343mg | Carbs 9.5g | Fiber 0.5g | Sugar 1.1g | Protein 10.4g

8. Ranch Chickpeas

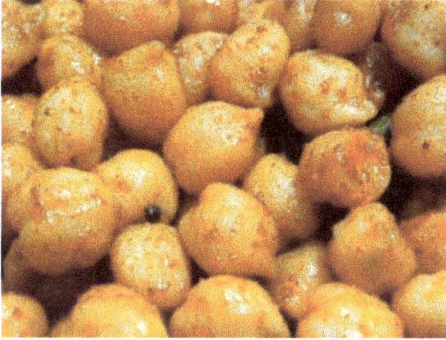

Prep Time: 10 minutes.
Cook Time: 8 minutes.
Serves: 4

Ingredients:

- 1 tablespoon dry ranch dressing
- 1 (15 ounces) can chickpeas, drained
- 2 tablespoons Buffalo wing sauce

Preparation:

1. At 350 degrees F, preheat your Ninja Air Fryer on Air Fry mode.
2. Drain the canned chickpeas and spread them on a baking sheet lined with a paper towel.
3. Toss the chickpeas with wing sauce and ranch dressing powder in a bowl.
4. Spread the chickpeas in the Air Fryer basket.
5. Return the Air Fryer basket to the Air Fryer and cook for 8 minutes.
6. Toss the chickpeas once cooked halfway through.
7. Serve warm.

Serving Suggestion: Serve with fresh yogurt dip or cucumber salad.

Variation Tip: Add hot sauce for seasoning.

Nutritional Information Per Serving:
Calories 186 | Fat 3g |Sodium 223mg | Carbs 31g | Fiber 8.7g | Sugar 5.5g | Protein 9.7g

9. Stuffed Mushrooms

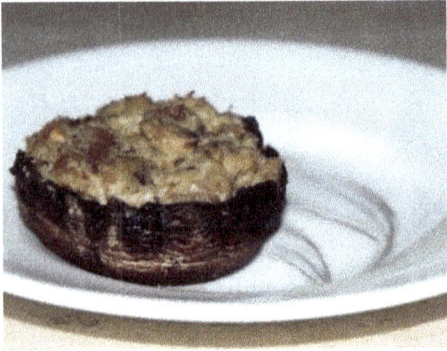

Prep Time: 15 minutes.

Cook Time: 8 minutes.

Serves: 6

Ingredients:

- 2 scallions, minced
- 4 ounces cream cheese, softened
- ¼ cup sharp Cheddar cheese, shredded
- ¼ teaspoon ground paprika
- 1 pinch salt
- 1 (16 ounces) package white button mushrooms
- Cooking spray

Preparation:

1. Destem the mushrooms and clean the caps.
2. At 360 degrees F, preheat your Ninja Air Fryer on Air Fry mode.
3. Whisk cream cheese with white parts of scallions, salt, and paprika in a small bowl.
4. Divide this filling in the mushroom caps.
5. Place half of the mushrooms in the Air Fryer basket and spray them with cooking spray.
6. Return the Air Fryer basket to the Air Fryer and for 8 minutes.
7. Cook the remaining mushroom in the same way.
8. Garnish with green parts from the scallions.
9. Serve warm.

Serving Suggestion: Serve with mayonnaise or cream cheese dip.

Variation Tip: Drizzle breadcrumbs on top before Air Frying.

Nutritional Information Per Serving:

Calories 103 | Fat 8.4g |Sodium 117mg | Carbs 3.5g | Fiber 0.9g | Sugar 1.5g | Protein 5.1g

10. Korean Chicken Wings

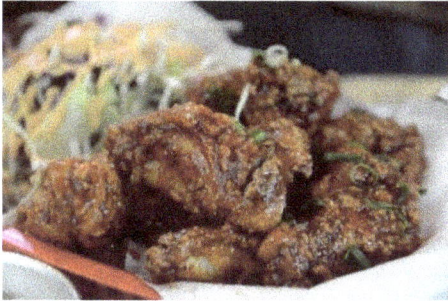

Prep Time: 10 minutes.
Cook Time: 15 minutes.
Serves: 8

Ingredients:

Sauce:

- ¼ cup hot honey
- 3 tablespoons gochujang
- 1 tablespoon brown sugar
- 1 tablespoon soy sauce
- 1 teaspoon lemon juice
- 2 teaspoons minced garlic
- 1 teaspoon fresh ginger root, minced
- ½ teaspoon salt
- ¼ teaspoon black pepper
- ¼ cup green onions, chopped

Wings:

- 2 pounds of chicken wings
- 1 teaspoon salt
- 1 teaspoon garlic powder
- 1 teaspoon onion powder
- ½ teaspoon black pepper
- ½ cup cornstarch

Garnish:

- 2 tablespoons green onions, chopped
- 1 teaspoon sesame seeds

Preparation:

1. Mix gochujang with hot honey, soy sauce, brown sugar, ginger, garlic, black pepper, salt, and lemon juice in a saucepan.

2. Place this saucepan on medium heat and cook for 5 minutes. on a simmer.
3. Stir in green onions, then remove from the heat.
4. At 400 degrees F, preheat your Ninja Air Fryer on Air Fry mode.
5. Mix garlic powder, onion powder, cornstarch, black pepper, and salt in a large bowl.
6. Spread the wings in the Air Fryer basket, cook in batches if needed.
7. Return the Air Fryer basket to the Air Fryer and for 10 minutes.
8. Flip the wings once cooked halfway through.
9. Transfer the air fried wings to a large bowl and pour the prepared sauce on top.
10. Toss well and serve warm.

Serving Suggestion: Serve Asian coleslaw or creamed cabbage.

Variation Tip: Use maple syrup instead of honey.

Nutritional Information Per Serving:

Calories 307 | Fat 8.6g |Sodium 510mg | Carbs 22.2g | Fiber 1.4g | Sugar 13g | Protein 33.6g

11. Mozzarella Sticks

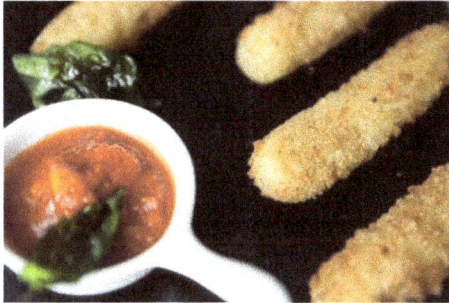

Prep Time: 15 minutes.
Cook Time: 12 minutes.
Serves: 6

Ingredients:

Batter:

- ½ cup of water
- ¼ cup all-purpose flour
- 5 tablespoons cornstarch
- 1 tablespoon cornmeal
- 1 teaspoon garlic powder
- ½ teaspoon salt

Coating:

- 1 cup panko bread crumbs
- ½ teaspoon salt
- ½ teaspoon ground black pepper
- ½ teaspoon parsley flakes
- ½ teaspoon garlic powder
- ¼ teaspoon onion powder
- ¼ teaspoon dried oregano
- ¼ teaspoon dried basil
- 5 ounces mozzarella cheese, cut into 1/2-inch strips
- 1 tablespoon all-purpose flour
- Cooking spray

Preparation:

1. Mix flour with cornstarch, garlic powder, cornmeal, salt, and water in a shallow bowl until smooth.
2. In another bowl, mix panko, parsley, black pepper, salt, garlic powder, onion powder, basil, and oregano in another shallow bowl.
3. First, the mozzarella sticks in the flour batter, then coat them with panko mixture.

4. Place the coated sticks in the Air Fryer basket.
5. Return the Air Fryer basket to the Air Fryer.
6. Select the Air Fry mode at 400 degrees F for 12 minutes.
7. Flip the sticks once cooked halfway through using a tong.
8. Serve warm.

Serving Suggestion: Serve with chunky red salsa.

Variation Tip: Use crushed cornflakes for breading to have extra crisp.

Nutritional Information Per Serving:

Calories 284 | Fat 7.9g |Sodium 704mg | Carbs 38.1g | Fiber 1.9g | Sugar 1.9g | Protein 14.8g

Chapter 3: Vegetables and Sides Recipes

1. Fried Tofu

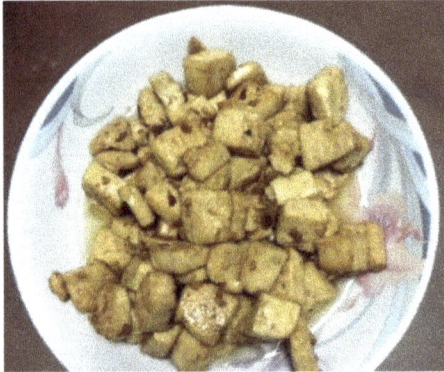

Prep Time: 10 minutes.

Cook Time: 15 minutes.

Serves: 4

Ingredients:

- 1 16-oz block tofu
- 2 tablespoons soy sauce
- 1 tablespoon toasted sesame oil
- 1 tablespoon olive oil
- 1 garlic clove, minced

Preparation:

1. Place the tofu block in between two heavy plates for 15 minutes. to squeeze the water.
2. Pat the tofu dry, dice it into small cubes then transfer to a suitable bowl.
3. Mix soy sauce, sesame oil, olive oil, and garlic in a small bowl.
4. Pour over the tofu cubes, mix and let them marinate for 15 minutes.
5. Drain the marinated tofu and place them in the Air Fryer basket.
6. Return the Air Fryer basket to the Air Fryer.
7. Select the Air Fry mode at 375 degrees F for 15 minutes.
8. Toss the tofu cubes once cooked halfway through, then resume cooking.
9. Serve warm.

Serving Suggestion: Serve with sautéed green vegetables.

Variation Tip: Add sautéed onion and carrot to the tofu cubes.

Nutritional Information Per Serving:

Calories 284 | Fat 7.9g |Sodium 704mg | Carbs 38.1g | Fiber 1.9g | Sugar 1.9g | Protein 14.8g

2. Kale Potato Nuggets

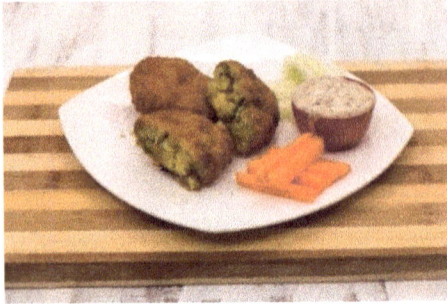

Prep Time: 15 minutes.
Cook Time: 18 minutes.
Serves: 4

Ingredients:

- 2 cups potatoes, chopped
- 1 teaspoon olive oil
- 1 garlic clove, minced
- 4 cups kale, chopped
- 1/8 cup almond milk
- 1/4 teaspoon sea salt
- 1/8 teaspoon ground black pepper
- Vegetable oil spray as needed

Preparation:

1. Set a cooking pot filled with water over medium heat.
2. Add potatoes to this boiling water and cook for 30 minutes. until soft.
3. Meanwhile, sauté garlic with oil in a skillet over medium-high heat until golden.
4. Stir in kale and sauté for 3 minutes., then transfer this mixture to a bowl.
5. Drain the boiled potatoes and add them to the kale.
6. Mix the potatoes with a potato masher.
7. Stir in salt, black pepper, and milk them, mix well.
8. Make 1-inch potato nuggets out of this mixture.
9. Place these nuggets in the Air Fryer basket.
10. Return the Air Fryer basket to the Air Fryer.
11. Select the Air Fry mode at 390 degrees F for 15 minutes.
12. Flip the nuggets once cooked halfway through, then resume cooking.
13. Serve warm.

Serving Suggestion: Serve with onion dip and sautéed carrots.

Variation Tip: Use breadcrumbs for breading to have extra crisp.

Nutritional Information Per Serving:

Calories 113 | Fat 3g |Sodium 152mg | Carbs 20g | Fiber 3g | Sugar 1.1g | Protein 3.5g

3. Air Fried Falafel

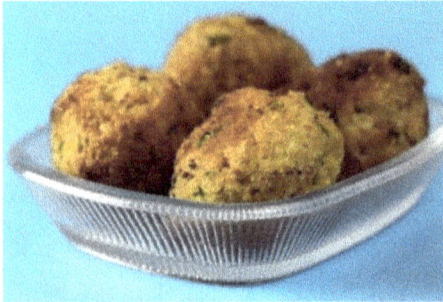

Prep Time: 15 minutes.

Cook Time: 10 minutes.

Serves: 6

Ingredients:

- 1 ½ cups dry garbanzo beans
- ½ cup fresh parsley, chopped
- ½ cup fresh cilantro, chopped
- ½ cup white onion, chopped
- 7 garlic cloves, minced
- 2 tablespoons all-purpose flour
- ½ teaspoons sea salt
- 1 tablespoon ground cumin
- ⅛ teaspoons ground cardamom
- 1 teaspoon ground coriander
- ⅛ teaspoons cayenne pepper

Preparation:

1. Soak garbanzo beans in a bowl filled with water for 24 hours.
2. Drain and transfer the beans to a cooking pot filled with water.
3. Cook the beans for 1 hour or more on simmer until soft.
4. Add cilantro, onion, garlic, and parsley to a food processor and blend until finely chopped.
5. Drain the cooked garbanzo beans and transfer them to the food processor.
6. Add salt, cardamom, cayenne, coriander, cumin, and flour.
7. Blend until it makes a rough dough.
8. Transfer this falafel mixture to a bowl, cover with a plastic wrap and refrigerate for 2 hours.
9. Make 1 ½ inches balls out of this bean's mixture.
10. Lightly press the balls and place them in the Air Fryer basket.
11. Return the Air Fryer basket to the Air Fryer.
12. Select the Air Fry mode at 400 degrees F for 10 minutes.
13. Flip the falafels once cooked halfway through the resume cooking.

14. Serve warm.

Serving Suggestion: Serve with tomato sauce or ketchup.

Variation Tip: Use crushed cornflakes for breading to have extra crisp.

Nutritional Information Per Serving:

Calories 206 | Fat 3.4g |Sodium 174mg | Carbs 35g | Fiber 9.4g | Sugar 5.9g | Protein 10.6g

4. Veggie Bites

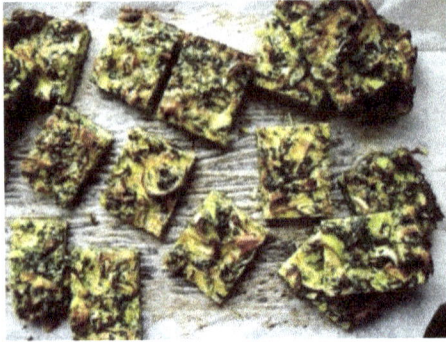

Prep Time: 10 minutes.
Cook Time: 45 minutes.
Serves: 6

Ingredients:

- 1 large broccoli, cut into florets
- 6 large carrots, diced
- Handful of garden peas
- ½ cauliflower, riced
- 1 large onion, peeled and diced
- 1 small courgette, diced
- 2 leeks, sliced
- 1 can coconut milk
- 2 oz. plain flour
- 1 cm cube ginger peeled and grated
- 1 tablespoon garlic puree
- 1 tablespoon olive oil
- 1 tablespoon Thai green curry paste
- 1 tablespoon coriander
- 1 tablespoon mixed spice
- 1 teaspoon cumin
- Salt and black pepper, to taste

Preparation:

1. Place leek and courgette in a steamer basket and steam them for 20 minutes.
2. Sauté onion, ginger, and garlic with olive oil in a skillet until soft.
3. Add steamed leek and courgette to the skillet and sauté for 5 minutes.
4. Stir in coconut milk and the rest of the spices.
5. Mix well, then add the cauliflower rice then cook for 10 minutes.
6. Remove the hot skillet from the heat and allow it to cool.
7. Cover and refrigerate this mixture for 1 hour.

8. Slice the mixture into bite-sized pieces and place these pieces in the Air Fryer basket.
9. Return the Air Fryer basket to the Air Fryer.
10. Select the Air Fry mode at 350 degrees F for 10 minutes.
11. Carefully flip the bites once cooked halfway through, then resume cooking.
12. Serve warm.

Serving Suggestion: Serve with mayonnaise or cream cheese dip.

Variation Tip: Add shredded brussels sprouts to the veggie mixture.

Nutritional Information Per Serving:

Calories 270 | Fat 14.6g |Sodium 394mg | Carbs 31.3g | Fiber 7.5g | Sugar 9.7g | Protein 6.4g

5. Parmesan Eggplant

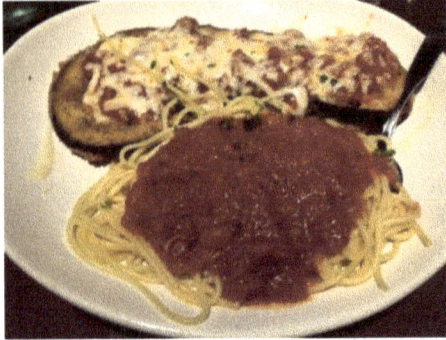

Prep Time: 15 minutes.
Cook Time: 15 minutes.
Serves: 4

Ingredients:

- 1/2 cup flour
- 1/2 cup almond milk
- 1/2 cup panko bread crumbs
- 2 tablespoons parmesan, grated
- Onion powder to taste
- Garlic powder to taste
- 1 large eggplant, stems removed and sliced
- Salt and black pepper, to taste

Eggplant parmesan:

- 1 cup marinara sauce
- 1/2 cup mozzarella shreds
- Parmesan, grated

Preparation:

1. Mix panko crumbs with garlic powder, black pepper, salt, onion powder, and vegan parmesan in a bowl.
2. First coat the eggplant slices with flour, then dip in the almond milk and finally coat with bread crumbs mixture.
3. Place the coated eggplant slices in the Air Fryer basket.
4. Return the Air Fryer basket to the Air Fryer.
5. Select the Air Fry mode at 390 degrees F for 15 minutes.
6. Flip the eggplant slices once cooked halfway through.
7. Place the eggplant slices on the serving plate and top them with marinara sauce and cheese.
8. Serve warm.

Serving Suggestion: Serve boiled spaghetti and marinara sauce on top of the side.

Variation Tip: Drizzle crushed crackers on top.

Nutritional Information Per Serving:
Calories 231 | Fat 9g |Sodium 271mg | Carbs 32.8g | Fiber 6.4g | Sugar 7g | Protein 6.3g

6. Potato Cakes

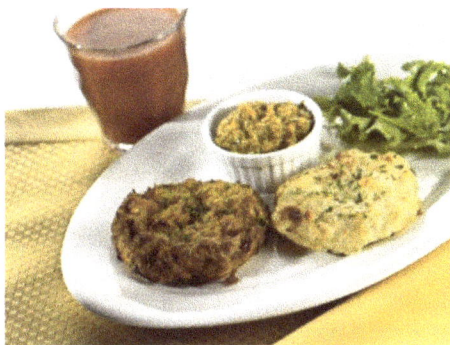

Prep Time: 10 minutes.
Cook Time: 35 minutes.
Serves: 4

Ingredients:

- 4 cups potatoes, diced
- 1 bunch green onions, chopped
- 1 lime, zest, and juice
- 1½ inch knob of fresh ginger
- 1 tablespoon tamari
- 4 tablespoons red curry paste
- 4 sheets nori, chopped
- 1 can heart of palm, drained
- ¾ cup canned artichoke hearts, drained
- Black pepper, to taste
- Salt, to taste

Preparation:

1. Add potato cubes to a pot filled with water.
2. Place it over medium heat and cook until potatoes are soft.
3. Drain the potatoes and transfer them to a suitable bowl.
4. Mash the potatoes with a masher, then add green onions, lime juice, and remaining ingredients.
5. Mix well and stir in artichoke shreds.

6. Stir well and make 4 patties out of this mixture.
7. Place the patties in the Air Fryer basket.
8. Return the Air Fryer basket to the Air Fryer.
9. Select the Air Fry mode at 375 degrees F for 10 minutes.
10. Flip the patties once cooked halfway through and resume cooking.
11. Serve warm.

Serving Suggestion: Serve with chunky red salsa or ketchup.

Variation Tip: Coat the cakes with breadcrumbs for extra crisp.

Nutritional Information Per Serving:

Calories 208 | Fat 5g |Sodium 1205mg | Carbs 34.1g | Fiber 7.8g | Sugar 2.5g | Protein 5.9g

7. Black Bean Burger

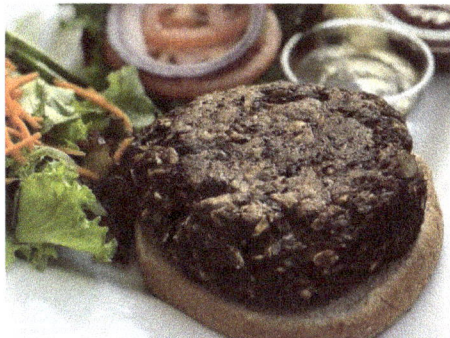

Prep Time: 15 minutes.
Cook Time: 15 minutes.
Serves: 6

Ingredients:

- 1 1/3 cups rolled oats
- 16 ounces canned black bean
- 3/4 cup salsa
- 1 tablespoon soy sauce
- 1 1/4 teaspoon mild chili powder
- 1/4-1/2 teaspoon chipotle Chile powder
- 1/2 teaspoon garlic powder
- 1/2 cup corn kernels

Preparation:

1. Add all the rolled oats to a food processor and pulse to get a coarse meal.
2. Add black beans, salsa, soy sauce, chili powder, Chile powder, and garlic powder.
3. Blend again for 1 minute, then transfer to a bowl.
4. Stir in corn kernel, then make six patties out of this mixture.
5. Place the black bean patties in the Air Fryer basket.
6. Return the Air Fryer basket to the Air Fryer.
7. Select the Air Fry mode at 375 degrees F for 15 minutes.
8. Flip the patties once cooked halfway through and resume cooking.
9. Serve warm.

Serving Suggestion: Serve with burger buns, lettuce leaves, and tomato slices along with mayonnaise or cream cheese dip.

Variation Tip: Add chopped onion and parsley to the bean's mixture.

Nutritional Information Per Serving:
Calories 350 | Fat 2.6g |Sodium 358mg | Carbs 64.6g | Fiber 14.4g | Sugar 3.3g | Protein 19.9g

8. Fried Mushrooms

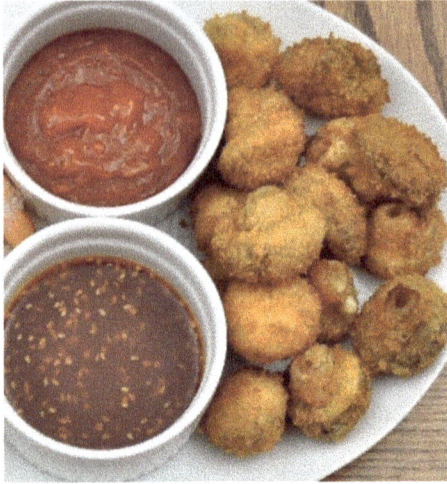

Prep Time: 15 minutes.
Cook Time: 25 minutes.
Serves: 6

Ingredients:

- 2 cups oyster mushrooms
- 1 cup buttermilk
- 1 ½ cups all-purpose flour
- 1 teaspoon salt
- 1 teaspoon black pepper
- 1 teaspoon garlic powder
- 1 teaspoon onion powder
- 1 teaspoon smoked paprika
- 1 teaspoon cumin
- 1 tablespoon oil

Preparation:

1. At 375 degrees F, preheat your Ninja Air Fryer on Air Fry mode.
2. Clean the mushrooms and then soak them in buttermilk for 15 minutes.
3. Mix all-purpose flour with onion powder, garlic powder, black pepper, salt, smoked paprika, and cumin in a suitable bowl.
4. Coat the mushrooms with flour mixture and then dip again with buttermilk.
5. Coat the mushrooms again with flour and buttermilk.
6. Place the coated mushrooms in the Air Fryer basket.
7. Return the Air Fryer basket to the Air Fryer and cook for 10 minutes.
8. Flip the mushrooms once cooked halfway through.
9. Serve warm.

Serving Suggestion: Serve with red chunky salsa or chili sauce.

Variation Tip: Use crushed cornflakes for breading to have extra crisp.

Nutritional Information Per Serving:

Calories 166 | Fat 3.2g |Sodium 437mg | Carbs 28.8g | Fiber 1.8g | Sugar 2.7g | Protein 5.8g

9. Veggie Wontons

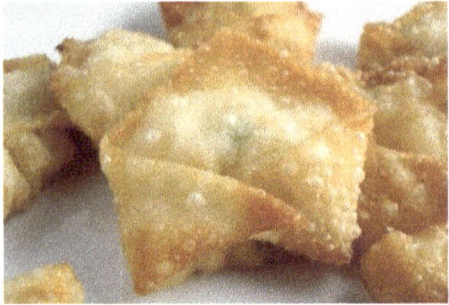

Prep Time: 15 minutes.
Cook Time: 8 minutes.
Serves: 15

Ingredients:

- 30 wonton wrappers
- 3/4 cup cabbage, grated
- 1/2 cup white onion, grated
- 1/2 cup carrot, grated
- 1/2 cup mushrooms, chopped
- 3/4 cup red pepper, chopped
- 1 tablespoon chili sauce
- 1 teaspoon garlic powder
- 1/2 teaspoon white pepper
- Pinch of salt
- 1/4 cup water
- Spray Olive Oil

Preparation:

1. Sauté cabbage, onion, carrot, mushrooms, and red pepper with olive oil in a skillet until soft.
2. Mix chili sauce, white pepper, salt, and garlic powder, then pour in the vegetables.
3. Stir and cook for 2 minutes. until well mixed.
4. Remove the filling from the heat and allow it cool.
5. Spread the wonton wrappers on the working surface.
6. Add 1 tablespoon of vegetable filling on top of each wrapper.
7. Wet their edges, then fold each wrapper in half and roll them in a wonton.
8. Place the wrapped wontons in the Air Fryer basket.
9. Return the Air Fryer basket to the Air Fryer.
10. Select the Air Fry mode at 320 degrees F for 6 minutes.
11. Serve warm.

Serving Suggestion: Serve with red chunky salsa or chili sauce.

Variation Tip: Add ground chicken to the filling.

Nutritional Information Per Serving:

Calories 193 | Fat 1g |Sodium 395mg | Carbs 38.7g | Fiber 1.6g | Sugar 0.9g | Protein 6.6g

10. General Tso's Cauliflower

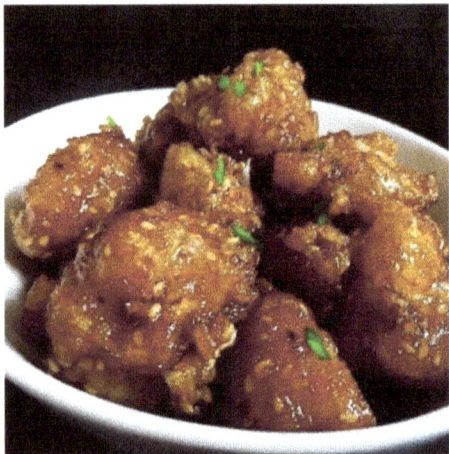

Prep Time: 15 minutes.
Cook Time: 28 minutes.
Serves:4

Ingredients:

Cauliflower

- ½ head cauliflower, cut into florets
- ½ cup flour
- 2 large eggs, whisked
- 1 cup panko breadcrumbs
- ¼ teaspoons salt
- ¼ teaspoons black pepper

General Tso's sauce

- 1 tablespoon sesame oil
- 2 garlic cloves, minced
- 1 tablespoon fresh ginger, grated
- ½ cup vegetable broth
- ¼ cup of soy sauce
- ¼ cup of rice vinegar
- ¼ cup brown sugar
- 2 tablespoons tomato paste
- 2 tablespoons cornstarch
- 2 tablespoons cold water

Preparation:

1. At 400 degrees F, preheat your Ninja Air Fryer on Air Fry mode.

2. Whisk egg in one bowl, spread panko in another bowl, and add flour to another bowl.
3. Dredge the cauliflower through the flour, dip in the egg and then coat with breadcrumbs.
4. Place the prepared cauliflower florets in the Air Fryer basket.
5. Return the Air Fryer basket to the Air Fryer and cook for 20 minutes.
6. Flip the florets once cooked halfway through, then resume cooking.
7. Meanwhile, sauté ginger, garlic, and sesame oil in a saucepan for 2 minutes.
8. Stir in the rest of the sauce ingredients except cornstarch.
9. Mix cornstarch with 2 tablespoons water in a bowl.
10. Pour the slurry into the sauce, mix and cook until the sauce thickens.
11. Remove the sauce from the heat and allow it to cool.
12. Toss in the baked cauliflower and mix well to coat.
13. Serve warm.

Serving Suggestion: Serve with boiled rice or noodles

Variation Tip: Use crushed cornflakes for breading to have extra crisp.

Nutritional Information Per Serving:

Calories 288 | Fat 6.9g |Sodium 761mg | Carbs 46g | Fiber 4g | Sugar 12g | Protein 9.6g

11. Garlic Mogo Chips

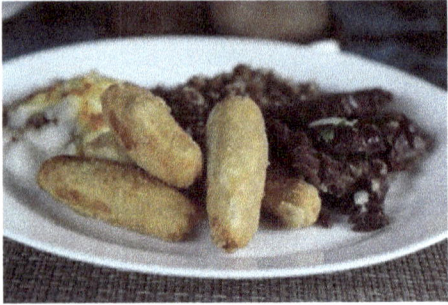

Prep Time: 20 minutes.
Cook Time: 25 minutes.
Serves: 4

Ingredients:

Mogo chips

- 1 lb. Mogo chips
- Salt to taste
- 1/2 teaspoon turmeric powder
- 1/2 teaspoon garlic powder
- 1 tablespoon lime juice
- 1/2 teaspoon oil
- 8 cups of water

Masala mix

- 1 teaspoon red chili powder
- Pinch dried chili flakes
- 1/2 teaspoon garlic powder
- Salt to taste
- 1 teaspoon lime juice
- 1/2 teaspoon lime zest
- 1 teaspoon oil

Preparation:

1. Mix water with oil, lime juice, turmeric powder, garlic powder, and salt in a saucepan.
2. Stir in Mogo chips and cook for 8-10 minutes. until the chips are boiled.
3. Drain and allow the chips to cool.
4. Mix all the spices for masala mix in a suitable bowl.
5. Toss in Mogo chips and mix well to coat.
6. Spread the chips in the Air Fryer basket.
7. Return the Air Fryer basket to the Air Fryer.

8. Select the Air Fry mode at 400 degrees F for 5 minutes.
9. Toss the chips once cooked halfway through, then resume cooking.
10. Serve warm.

Serving Suggestion: Serve with red chunky salsa or chili sauce.

Variation Tip: Use crushed cornflakes for breading to have extra crisp.

Nutritional Information Per Serving:

Calories 212 | Fat 11.8g |Sodium 321mg | Carbs 24.6g | Fiber 4.4g | Sugar 8g | Protein 7.3g

Chapter 4: Fish and Seafood Recipes

1. Fried Masala Fish

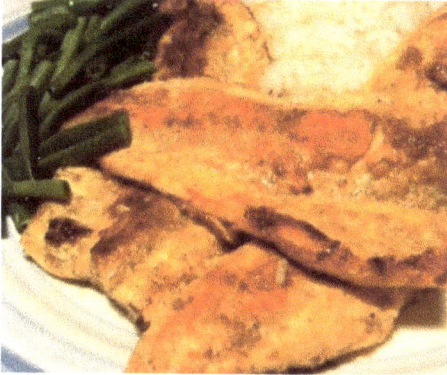

Prep Time: 15 minutes.
Cook Time: 10 minutes.
Serves: 4

Ingredients:

- 2 pounds fish fillets
- 4 tablespoons olive oil
- 3/4 teaspoon turmeric
- 1 teaspoon cayenne pepper
- 1 teaspoon salt
- 1 tablespoon fenugreek leaves
- 1 ½ teaspoon freshly ground cumin
- 2 teaspoons amchur powder
- 2 tablespoons ground almonds

To finish

- Extra lemon juice
- Chopped coriander leaves
- Sliced almonds

Preparation:

1. Mix turmeric with fenugreek leaves, almond ground, amchur powder, cumin, salt, and cayenne pepper in a small bow.
2. Place the prepared fish fillets in a tray and rub it with the spice mixture.
3. Marinate for 15 minutes., then place the fish in the Air Fryer basket.
4. Return the Air Fryer basket to the Air Fryer.

5. Select the Air Fry mode at 450 degrees F for 10 minutes.
6. Garnish with lemon juice, cilantro, and almond slices.
7. Serve.

Serving Suggestion: Serve with sautéed green beans or asparagus.

Variation Tip: Rub the fish with lemon juice before seasoning.

Nutritional Information Per Serving:

Calories 260 | Fat 16g |Sodium 585mg | Carbs 3.1g | Fiber 1.3g | Sugar 0.2g | Protein 25.5g

2. Southern Fried Catfish

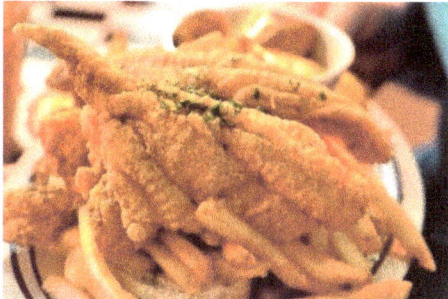

Prep Time: 15 minutes.
Cook Time: 20 minutes.
Serves: 2

Ingredients:

- Cooking spray
- 1 teaspoon light brown sugar
- ½ teaspoon crushed red pepper
- ⅜ teaspoon kosher salt, divided
- 2 -6 ounces catfish fillets
- ¼ cup all-purpose flour
- 1 large egg, beaten
- ⅓ cup panko bread crumbs
- 12 ounces fresh green beans, trimmed
- ¼ teaspoon black pepper

Preparation:

1. Toss green beans with brown sugar, salt, and red pepper in a bowl
2. Spread the green beans in the Air Fryer basket and spray it with cooking oil.
3. Return the Air Fryer basket to the Air Fryer.
4. Select the Air Fry mode at 400 degrees F for 12 minutes.
5. Transfer the green beans to a bowl and cover with aluminum foil.
6. Spread the panko crumbs in one plate, beat the egg in a bowl, and spread flour in a bowl.
7. Coat the fish with the flour, dip in the egg, and coat with the crumbs.
8. Place the fish in the Air Fryer basket and spray with cooking spray.
9. Return the Air Fryer basket to the Air Fryer.
10. Select the Air Fry mode at 400 degrees F for 8 minutes.
11. Season the air fried fish with black pepper and salt.
12. Garnish with green beans.
13. Serve warm.

Serving Suggestion: Serve with crispy potato fries.

Variation Tip: Use crushed cornflakes for breading to have extra crisp.

Nutritional Information Per Serving:

Calories 266 | Fat 6.3g |Sodium 193mg | Carbs 39.1g | Fiber 7.2g | Sugar 5.2g | Protein 14.8g

3. Popcorn Shrimp

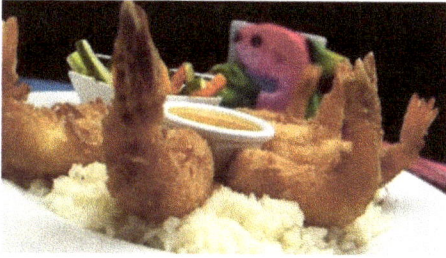

Prep Time: 20 minutes.

Cook Time: 8 minutes.

Serves: 4

Ingredients:

- ½ cup all-purpose flour
- 2 eggs, beaten
- 2 tablespoons water
- 1 ½ cups panko breadcrumbs
- 1 tablespoon ground cumin
- 1 tablespoon garlic powder
- 1-pound small shrimp, peeled and deveined
- ½ cup ketchup
- 2 tablespoons chipotle chiles in adobo, chopped
- 2 tablespoons fresh cilantro, chopped
- 2 tablespoons lime juice
- ⅛ teaspoon kosher salt

Preparation:

1. Beat eggs with water in one bowl, and mix panko with garlic powder and cumin in another bowl.
2. Coat the shrimp with the flour, dip them in the eggs then coat with panko mixture.
3. Spread the shrimp in the greased Air Fryer basket.
4. Return the Air Fryer basket to the Air Fryer.
5. Select the Air Fry mode at 360 degrees F for 8 minutes.
6. Toss the shrimp once cooked halfway through and resume cooking.
7. Mix ketchup with the rest of the ingredients in a suitable bowl.
8. Serve the shrimp with the sauce.

Serving Suggestion: Serve on top of mashed potato or mashed cauliflower.

Variation Tip: Use crushed cornflakes for breading to have extra crisp.

Nutritional Information Per Serving:

Calories 297 | Fat 1g |Sodium 291mg | Carbs 35g | Fiber 1g | Sugar 9g | Protein 29g

4. Scallops with Herb Sauce

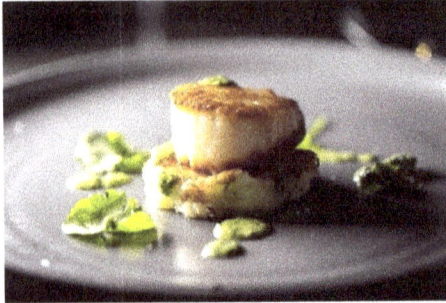

Prep Time: 15 minutes.
Cook Time: 6 minutes.
Serves: 2

Ingredients:

- 8 large sea scallops, cleaned
- ¼ teaspoon ground black pepper
- ⅛ teaspoon salt
- Cooking spray
- ¼ cup olive oil
- 2 tablespoons parsley, chopped
- 2 teaspoons capers, chopped
- 1 teaspoon lemon zest, grated
- ½ teaspoon garlic, chopped
- Lemon wedges

Preparation:

1. Season cleaned scallops with salt and black pepper.
2. Place the prepared scallops in the Air Fryer basket and spray them with cooking oil.
3. Return the Air Fryer basket to the Air Fryer.
4. Select the Air Fry mode at 400 degrees F for 6 minutes.
5. Meanwhile, mix capers, parsley, oil, garlic, and lemon zest in a small bowl.
6. Serve the scallops with capers mixture.
7. Enjoy.

Serving Suggestion: Serve with sautéed or fresh greens with melted butter.

Variation Tip: Wrap the scallops in the bacon slices before cooking.

Nutritional Information Per Serving:
Calories 348 | Fat 30g |Sodium 660mg | Carbs 5g | Fiber 0g | Sugar 0g | Protein 14g

5. Breaded Scallops

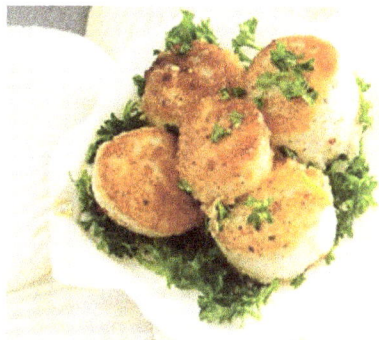

Prep Time: 10 minutes.
Cook Time: 5 minutes.
Serves: 4

Ingredients:

- ½ cup buttery crackers, crushed
- ½ teaspoon garlic powder
- ½ teaspoon seafood seasoning
- 2 tablespoons butter, melted
- 1-pound sea scallops
- Cooking spray

Preparation:

1. At 390 degrees F, preheat your Ninja Air Fryer on Air Fry mode.
2. Mix seafood seasoning, garlic powder, and cracker crumbs in a bowl.
3. Add melted butter to a bowl and keep it aside.
4. Dip the scallops in the melted butter and then coat with the breading.
5. Spread the scallops in the Air Fryer basket and spray with cooking spray.
6. Return the Air Fryer basket to the Air Fryer and cook for 4 minutes.
7. Flip the scallops once cooked halfway through and resume cooking.
8. Serve.

Serving Suggestion: Serve on a bed of freshly chopped parsley leaves.

Variation Tip: Use crushed cornflakes for breading to have extra crisp.

Nutritional Information Per Serving:
Calories 257 | Fat 10.4g | Sodium 431mg | Carbs 20g | Fiber 0g | Sugar 1.6g | Protein 21g

6. Fish Cakes

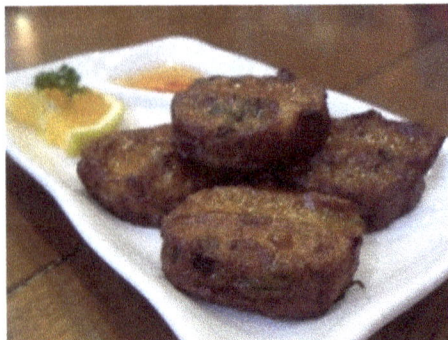

Prep Time: 15 minutes.
Cook Time: 10 minutes.
Serves: 4

Ingredients:

- Cooking spray
- 10 ounces white fish, chopped
- ⅔ cup panko breadcrumbs
- 3 tablespoons fresh cilantro, chopped
- 2 tablespoons Thai sweet chili sauce
- 2 tablespoons mayonnaise
- 1 large egg
- ⅛ teaspoon salt
- ¼ teaspoon ground pepper
- 2 lime wedges

Preparation:

1. Mix fish with mayonnaise, chili sauce, cilantro, panko, salt, black pepper, and egg in a medium bowl.
2. Make 3 inches diameter fish cakes out of this mixture.
3. Place the cakes in the Air Fryer basket and spray them with cooking oil.
4. Return the Air Fryer basket to the Air Fryer.
5. Select the Air Fry mode at 400 degrees F for 10 minutes.
6. Flip the cakes once cooked halfway through.
7. Serve warm.

Serving Suggestion: Serve with chili sauce or tomato ketchup.

Variation Tip: Use the drained tuna instead of white fish.

Nutritional Information Per Serving:
Calories 399 | Fat 16g |Sodium 537mg | Carbs 28g | Fiber 3g | Sugar 10g | Protein 35g

7. Air-Fried Salmon

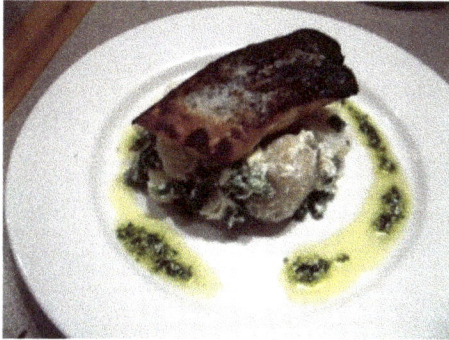 Prep Time: 10 minutes.
Cook Time: 15 minutes.
Serves: 2

Ingredients:

- Cooking spray
- 2 tablespoons horseradish, grated
- 1 tablespoon parsley, chopped
- 1 tablespoon capers, chopped
- 1 tablespoon olive oil
- 1-12-ounce skinless salmon fillet
- ¼ teaspoon salt
- ¼ teaspoon ground black pepper

Preparation:

1. Mix horseradish with capers, parsley, and oil in a small bowl.
2. Season the salmon with black pepper and salt.
3. Place the salmon in the Air Fryer basket and spread the horseradish mixture on top.
4. Return the Air Fryer basket to the Air Fryer.
5. Select the Air Fry mode at 375 degrees F for 15 minutes.
6. Serve warm.

Serving Suggestion: Serve with melted butter on top.

Variation Tip: Rub the salmon with lemon juice before cooking.

Nutritional Information Per Serving:
Calories 305 | Fat 15g |Sodium 482mg | Carbs 17g | Fiber 3g | Sugar 2g | Protein 35g

8. White Fish with Garlic

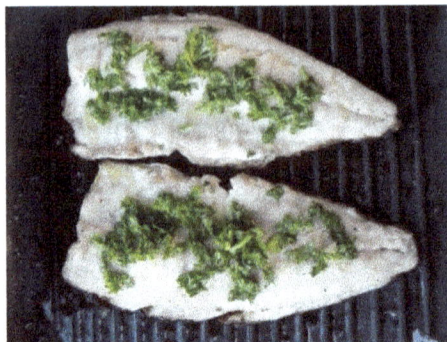

Prep Time: 10 minutes.
Cook Time: 12 minutes.
Serves: 2

Ingredients:

- 2 -6 ounces tilapia filets
- 1/2 teaspoon garlic powder
- 1/2 teaspoon lemon pepper seasoning
- 1/2 teaspoon onion powder
- Sea salt, to taste
- Black pepper, to taste
- Fresh chopped parsley
- Lemon wedges

Preparation:

1. At 360 degrees F, preheat your Ninja Air Fryer on Air Fry mode.
2. Coat the fish fillets with olive oil, lemon pepper, garlic powder, black pepper, salt, and onion powder.
3. Place the fish in the Air Fryer basket and top it with lemon wedges.
4. Return the Air Fryer basket to the Air Fryer.
5. Select the Air Fry mode at 360 degrees F for 12 minutes.
6. Garnish with parsley and lemon wedges.
7. Serve warm.

Serving Suggestion: Serve with melted butter on top.

Variation Tip: Rub the fish fillets with lemon juice before cooking.

Nutritional Information Per Serving:
Calories 336 | Fat 6g |Sodium 181mg | Carbs 1.3g | Fiber 0.2g | Sugar 0.4g | Protein 69.2g

9. Crab Cakes

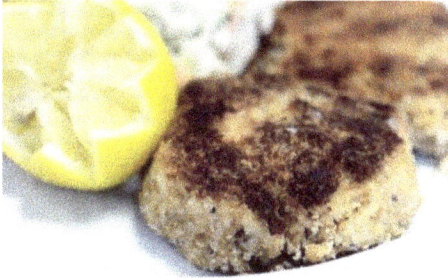

Prep Time: 15 minutes.

Cook Time: 10 minutes.

Serves: 6

Ingredients:

- 1 egg, beaten
- 2 tablespoons mayonnaise
- 1 teaspoon Worcestershire sauce
- 1 teaspoon Dijon mustard
- 1 teaspoon seafood seasoning
- ½ teaspoon hot pepper sauce
- 2 tablespoons green onion, chopped
- 1-pound crabmeat, drained
- 3 tablespoons milk
- Salt and black pepper, to taste
- 11 crackers saltine crackers, crushed
- 1 teaspoon baking powder
- 4 wedges lemon
- Olive oil cooking spray

Preparation:

1. Mix egg with mustard, spring onion, mayonnaise, Worcestershire sauce, hot pepper sauce and seafood seasoning in a small bowl.
2. Shred the crab meat in a medium bowl with a fork and stir in black pepper, salt and milk.
3. Mix and add baking powder, crushed saltines, and egg mixture.
4. Mix well and make 8 patties out of this mixture.
5. Place the patties in the Air Fryer basket.
6. Return the Air Fryer basket to the Air Fryer.
7. Select the Air Fry mode at 400 degrees F for 10 minutes.
8. Flip the cakes once cooked halfway through.
9. Serve warm.

Serving Suggestion: Enjoy with creamy coleslaw on the side.

Variation Tip: Use crushed cornflakes instead of saltines.

Nutritional Information Per Serving:

Calories 155 | Fat 4.2g |Sodium 963mg | Carbs 21.5g | Fiber 0.8g | Sugar 5.7g | Protein 8.1g

10. Lobster Tails with Garlic Butter

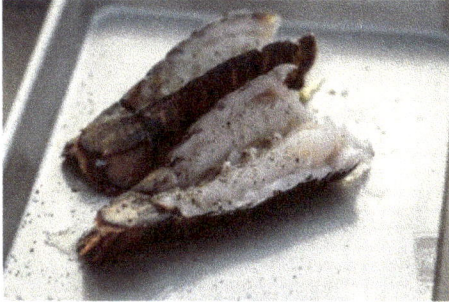

Prep Time: 15 minutes.

Cook Time: 8 minutes.

Serves: 2

Ingredients:

- 2 (4 ounces) lobster tails
- 4 tablespoons butter
- 1 teaspoon lemon zest
- 1 garlic clove, grated
- Salt and black pepper, to taste
- 1 teaspoon fresh parsley, chopped
- 2 wedges lemon

Preparation:

1. Spread the lobster tails into a butterfly by cutting the shell lengthwise.
2. Place the butterflied lobster tails in the Air Fryer basket.
3. Sauté garlic and lemon zest with butter in a saucepan for 30 seconds.
4. Brush the butter over the lobster tail and drizzle black pepper and salt on top.
5. Place the buttered lobster tail in the Air Fryer basket.
6. Return the Air Fryer basket to the Air Fryer.
7. Select the Air Fry mode at 380 degrees F for 7 minutes.
8. Garnish with remaining butter, parsley, and lemon wedges.
9. Serve warm.

Serving Suggestion: Serve with melted butter on top.

Variation Tip: Drizzle breadcrumbs on top before Air Frying.

Nutritional Information Per Serving:

Calories 308 | Fat 24g |Sodium 715mg | Carbs 0.8g | Fiber 0.1g | Sugar 0.1g | Protein 21.9g

11. Lobster Stuffed Mushrooms

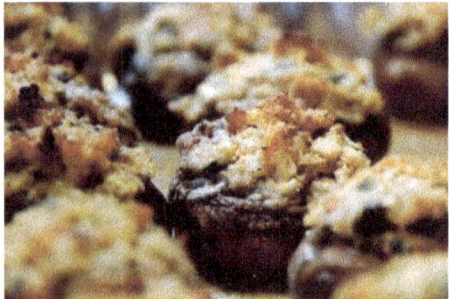

Prep Time: 20 minutes.
Cook Time: 15 minutes.
Serves: 5

Ingredients:

- 1 garlic clove, minced
- 1 celery stalk, chopped
- 1/2 red pepper, chopped
- 1 teaspoon old bay seasonings
- 1 egg
- 10 mushrooms caps
- 1 tablespoon olive oil
- 1/2 cup lobster meat, chopped
- 10 saltine crackers, crumbled
- 1 cup mozzarella cheese, shredded

Preparation:

1. Sauté celery, garlic, and pepper with olive oil in a pan for 5 minutes.
2. Stir in onion, garlic, seasoning, crushed cracker, and crab meat.
3. Add one egg, then mix well.
4. Divide the mixture into the mushroom caps.
5. Place the mushroom caps in the Air Fryer basket and drizzle cheese on top.
6. Return the Air Fryer basket to the Air Fryer.
7. Cook on Air Fry mode for 10 minutes. at 350 degrees F.
8. Serve warm.

Serving Suggestion: Serve with melted butter on top.

Variation Tip: Add crab meat to the filling.

Nutritional Information Per Serving:
Calories 196 | Fat 7.1g |Sodium 492mg | Carbs 21.6g | Fiber 2.9g | Sugar 0.8g | Protein 13.4g

12. Beer Battered Cod

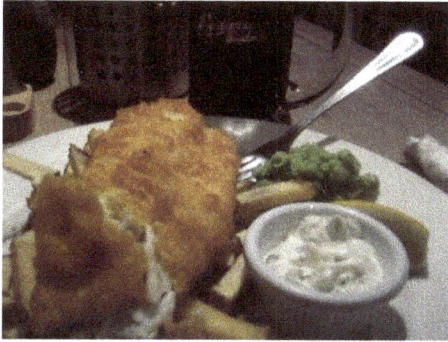

Prep Time: 15 minutes.
Cook Time: 12 minutes.
Serves: 4

Ingredients:

- 1 ¾ cup all-purpose flour
- 2 tablespoons cornstarch
- ½ teaspoon baking soda
- 6 ounces beer
- 1 egg beaten
- ½ teaspoon paprika
- 1 teaspoon salt
- ¼ teaspoon black pepper
- Pinch cayenne pepper
- 1½ pounds cod, cut into 4 pieces
- Vegetable oil

Preparation:

1. Mix baking soda, cornstarch, and 1 cup flour in a large bowl.
2. Stir in egg and beer, then mix well until smooth.
3. Cover the batter with a plastic sheet and refrigerate for 20 minutes.
4. Mix ¾ cup flour with cayenne pepper, black pepper, salt, and paprika in another bowl.
5. Coat the fish with the flour mixture, then dip it in the flour batter.
6. Place the fish in the Air Fryer basket and spray them with cooking oil.
7. Return the Air Fryer basket to the Air Fryer.
8. Select the Air Fry mode at 390 degrees F for 12 minutes.
9. Serve warm.

Serving Suggestion: Serve with creamy dip and crispy fries.

Variation Tip: Use crushed cornflakes for breading to have extra crisp.

Nutritional Information Per Serving:

Calories 275 | Fat 1.4g |Sodium 582mg | Carbs 31.5g | Fiber 1.1g | Sugar 0.1g | Protein 29.8g

Chapter 5: Poultry Mains Recipes

1. Paprika Chicken Wings

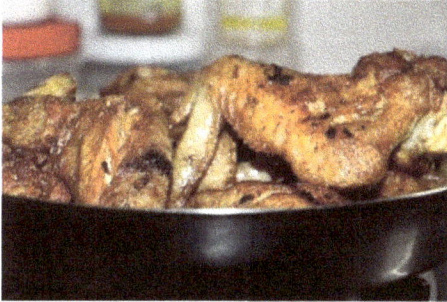

Prep Time: 15 minutes.
Cook Time: 24 minutes.
Serves: 6

Ingredients:

- 1 ½ lbs chicken wings
- 1/4 teaspoon sea salt
- 1/2 teaspoon black pepper
- 1/2 teaspoon smoked paprika
- 1/2 teaspoon garlic powder
- 1/2 teaspoon onion powder
- 1 tablespoon baking powder

Preparation:

1. Mix smoked paprika, black pepper, salt, garlic powder, baking powder, and onion powder in a small bowl.
2. Add all the chicken wings to a large bowl and drizzle the spice mixture over the wings.
3. Toss well and transfer the wings to an Air Fryer basket.
4. Return the Air Fryer basket to the Air Fryer.
5. Select the Air Fry mode at 400 degrees F for 24 minutes.
6. Toss the wings once cooked halfway through.
7. Serve warm.

Serving Suggestion: Serve with tomato ketchup or chili sauce.

Variation Tip: Dust the chicken with flour before seasoning.

Nutritional Information Per Serving:
Calories 220 | Fat 1.7g |Sodium 178mg | Carbs 1.7g | Fiber 0.2g | Sugar 0.2g | Protein 32.9g

2. Breaded Chicken Legs

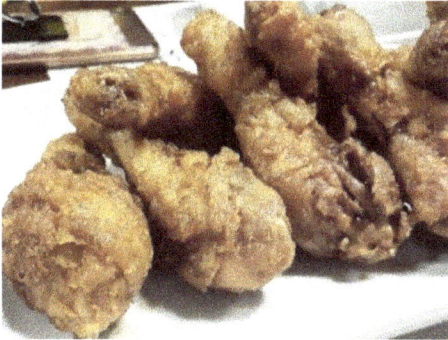

Prep Time: 20 minutes.
Cook Time: 24 minutes.
Serves: 6

Ingredients:

- 12 chicken legs
- 2 tablespoons seasoned salt
- 4 tablespoons olive oil
- 1 bag chicken breading

Preparation:

1. Toss drumsticks with olive oil and drizzle seasoning on top
2. Mix well to coat and coat the drumsticks with breadcrumbs.
3. Place the coated drumsticks in the Air Fryer basket and spray them with cooking oil.
4. Return the Air Fryer basket to the Air Fryer.
5. Select the Air Fry mode at 400 degrees F for 24 minutes.
6. Flip the drumsticks once cooked halfway through, then resume cooking.
7. Serve warm.

Serving Suggestion: Serve with tomato ketchup or chili sauce.

Variation Tip: Use crushed cornflakes for breading to have extra crisp.

Nutritional Information Per Serving:
Calories 380 | Fat 29g |Sodium 821mg | Carbs 34.6g | Fiber 0g | Sugar 0g | Protein 30g

3. Chicken Nuggets

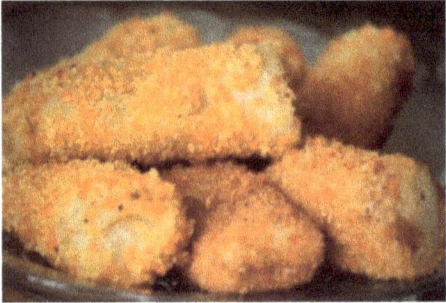

Prep Time: 15 minutes.

Cook Time:10 minutes.

Serves: 6

Ingredients:

- 1 ½ lbs chicken breasts, diced
- 1 tablespoon oil

Wet batter

- ½ cup of water cold
- 1 egg
- ¾ cup all-purpose flour sifted

Breadcrumbs

- 1 cup unseasoned breadcrumbs
- 1 teaspoon of sea salt
- ½ teaspoons cayenne pepper

Preparation:

1. Beat and whisk egg with water in a shallow bowl.
2. Stir in flour and mix well until it makes a smooth batter.
3. Mix breadcrumbs with cayenne pepper and salt in a shallow bowl.
4. Dip the chicken chunks in the batter and coat with the breadcrumbs.
5. Return the Air Fryer basket to the Air Fryer.
6. Select the Air Fry mode at 360 degrees F for 10 minutes.
7. Toss the chicken pieces once cooked halfway through and then resume cooking.
8. Serve warm.

Serving Suggestion: Serve with tomato ketchup or chili sauce.

Variation Tip: Use crushed cornflakes for breading to have extra crisp.

Nutritional Information Per Serving:

Calories 374 | Fat 13g |Sodium 552mg | Carbs 25g | Fiber 1.2g | Sugar 1.2g | Protein 37.7g

4. Greek Turkey Burgers

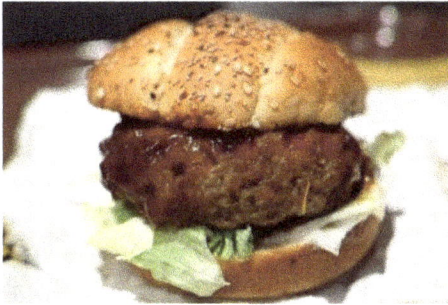

Prep Time: 20 minutes.
Cook Time: 15 minutes.
Serves: 2

Ingredients:

- 8 ounces of turkey ground
- 1 ½ tablespoon olive oil
- 2 teaspoons fresh oregano, chopped
- ½ teaspoon red pepper, crushed
- ¼ teaspoon salt
- 2 garlic cloves, grated
- ½ cup baby spinach leaves
- ¼ cup red onion, thinly sliced
- ½ tablespoon red-wine vinegar
- ¼ cup feta cheese, crumbled
- 2 whole-wheat burger buns, split and toasted

Preparation:

1. Mix turkey ground with oregano, oil, salt, garlic, and red pepper in a bowl.
2. Make 2 patties out of this mixture.
3. Place these patties in the Air Fryer basket and spray them with cooking oil.
4. Return the Air Fryer basket to the Air Fryer.
5. Select the Air Fry mode at 360 degrees F for 15 minutes.
6. Meanwhile, mix the onion with vinegar and spinach in a bowl.
7. Divide the spinach mixture into the burger buns, feta, and patties.
8. Serve warm.

Serving Suggestion: Serve with tomato ketchup or chili sauce.

Variation Tip: Use chicken ground instead of turkey ground.

Nutritional Information Per Serving:
Calories 351 | Fat 16g |Sodium 777mg | Carbs 26g | Fiber 4g | Sugar 5g | Protein 28g

5. Herbed Chicken Breast

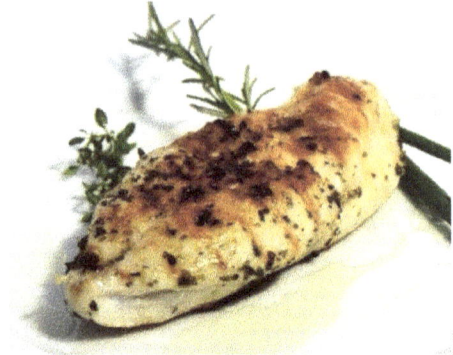

Prep Time: 15 minutes.
Cook Time: 22 minutes.
Serves: 4

Ingredients:

- Cooking spray
- 4 boneless skinless chicken breasts
- 1/2 teaspoon garlic powder
- 1/2 teaspoon salt
- 1/8 teaspoon black pepper
- 1/2 teaspoon dried oregano

Preparation:

1. Mix garlic powder, oregano, black pepper, and salt in a small bowl.
2. Spray the chicken breast with cooking spray.
3. Rub the chicken with the seasoning mix liberally.
4. Place the seasoned chicken breast in the Air Fryer basket.
5. Return the Air Fryer basket to the Air Fryer.
6. Select the Air Fry mode at 360 degrees F for 22 minutes.
7. Flip the chicken once cooked halfway through, drizzle the remaining seasoning.
8. Resume cooking and cook until the chicken is golden.
9. Serve warm.

Serving Suggestion: Serve with tomato ketchup or chili sauce.

Variation Tip: Rub the chicken with lemon juice before seasoning.

Nutritional Information Per Serving:

Calories 268 | Fat 10.4g |Sodium 411mg | Carbs 0.4g | Fiber 0.1g | Sugar 0.1g | Protein 40.6g

6. Tangy Chicken Drumsticks

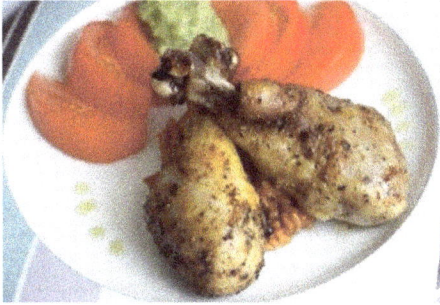

Prep Time: 15 minutes.

Cook Time: 20 minutes.

Serves: 4

Ingredients:

- 1 teaspoon paprika
- 8 chicken drumsticks
- 2 tablespoons olive oil
- 1 teaspoon of sea salt
- 1 teaspoon fresh cracked pepper
- 1 teaspoon garlic powder
- 1/2 teaspoon cumin

Preparation:

1. Mix and whisk all the spices and herbs in a small bowl.
2. Toss the drumsticks with olive oil and the spice mixture to coat well in a bowl.
3. At 400 degrees F, preheat your Ninja Air Fryer on Air Fry mode.
4. Spread the drumsticks in the Air Fryer basket.
5. Return the Air Fryer basket to the Air Fryer.
6. Select the Air Fry mode at 400 degrees F for 20 minutes.
7. Flip the drumsticks once cooked halfway through.
8. Serve warm.

Serving Suggestion: Serve with fresh-cut tomatoes and sautéed greens.

Variation Tip: Rub the chicken with lemon juice before seasoning.

Nutritional Information Per Serving:

Calories 220 | Fat 13g |Sodium 542mg | Carbs 0.9g | Fiber 0.3g | Sugar 0.2g | Protein 25.6g

7. Turkey Breast with Cherry Glaze

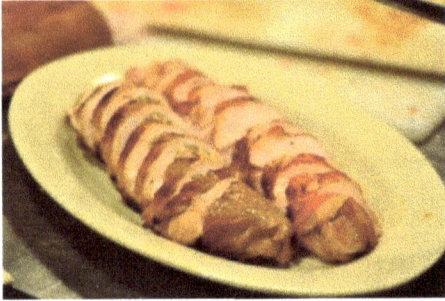

Prep Time: 15 minutes.
Cook Time: 42 minutes.
Serves: 10

Ingredients:

- 5 pounds bone-in turkey breast
- 1 teaspoon dried thyme
- ½ teaspoon dried sage
- 2 teaspoons olive oil
- 1 teaspoon salt
- ½ teaspoon black pepper
- ½ cup cherry preserves
- 1 tablespoon thyme leaves, chopped
- 1 teaspoon soy sauce
- Freshly ground black pepper, to taste

Preparation:

1. At 350 degrees F, preheat your Ninja Air Fryer on Air Fry mode.
2. Rub the turkey breast with olive oil, thyme, black pepper, sage, and salt.
3. Place the seasoned turkey breast in the Air Fryer basket.
4. Return the Air Fryer basket to the Air Fryer.
5. Select the Air Fry mode at 350 degrees F for 25 minutes.
6. Flip the turkey breast and continue cooking for another 12 minutes.
7. Meanwhile, mix cherry preserves with black pepper, soy sauce, and thyme in a saucepan.
8. Mix and cook for 5 minutes. until it makes a thick glaze.
9. Pour the glaze overcooked turkey breast.
10. Serve warm.

Serving Suggestion: Serve with warm corn tortilla and Greek salad.

Variation Tip: Coat and dust the turkey leg with flour before seasoning.

Nutritional Information Per Serving:

Calories 353 | Fat 5g |Sodium 818mg | Carbs 53.2g | Fiber 4.4g | Sugar 8g | Protein 17.3g

8. Thanksgiving Turkey Breasts

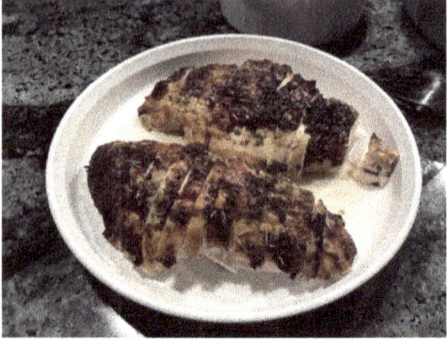

Prep Time: 10 minutes.

Cook Time: 35 minutes.

Serves: 4

Ingredients:

- 1 teaspoon kosher salt
- 1 teaspoon dried thyme
- 1 teaspoon ground rosemary
- 1/2 teaspoon black pepper
- 1/2 teaspoon dried sage
- 1/2 teaspoon garlic powder
- 1/2 teaspoon paprika
- 1/2 teaspoon dark brown sugar
- 1 bone-in, skin-on turkey breast
- Olive oil, for brushing

Preparation:

1. Mix garlic powder, sage, black pepper, rosemary, thyme, salt, brown sugar, and paprika in a small bowl.
2. Rub the prepared turkey breast with olive oil and spice mixture.
3. Place the turkey in a 3 ½ quart or bigger Air Fryer.
4. Return the Air Fryer basket to the Air Fryer.
5. Select the Roast mode at 400 degrees F for 20 minutes.
6. Flip the turkey and cook for another 15 minutes.
7. Slice and serve warm.

Serving Suggestion: Serve with tomato ketchup or chili sauce.

Variation Tip: Coat and dust the turkey breast with flour before seasoning.

Nutritional Information Per Serving:

Calories 346 | Fat 16.1g |Sodium 882mg | Carbs 1.3g | Fiber 0.5g | Sugar 0.5g | Protein 48.2g

9. Seasoned Turkey Leg

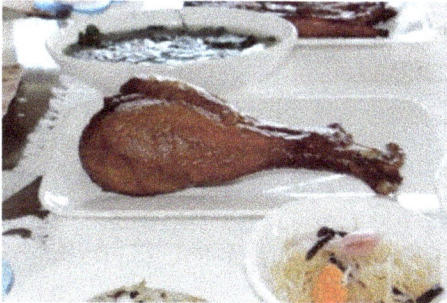

Prep Time: 10 minutes.
Cook Time: 27 minutes.
Serves: 2

Ingredients:

- 1 lb. turkey leg
- 1 teaspoon poultry seasoning
- 1 teaspoon garlic salt

Preparation:

1. Rub the turkey leg with poultry seasoning and garlic salt.
2. Place the turkey leg in the Air Fryer basket.
3. Return the Air Fryer basket to the Air Fryer.
4. Select the Air Fry mode at 350 degrees F for 27 minutes.
5. Flip the turkey leg once cooked halfway through.
6. Serve warm.

Serving Suggestion: Serve with warm corn tortilla and Greek salad.

Variation Tip: Coat and dust the turkey leg with flour before seasoning.

Nutritional Information Per Serving:
Calories 502 | Fat 25g |Sodium 230mg | Carbs 1.5g | Fiber 0.2g | Sugar 0.4g | Protein 64.1g

10. Chinese Roasted Duck

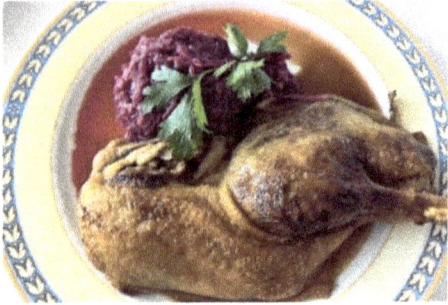

Prep Time: 20 minutes.
Cook Time: 52 minutes.
Serves: 4

Ingredients:

- 2 lbs of frozen rice duck
- 1 tablespoon hoisin sauce
- 1 teaspoon five spices powder
- 1 teaspoon black pepper
- 2 tablespoons Shaoxing wine
- 1 tablespoon sugar
- 1 teaspoon salt
- 1 tablespoon Sichuan peppercorn
- 4-star anise
- 4 cinnamon sticks
- 1 spring onion, chopped
- 2 slices ginger
- 4 cups of water

honey wash:

- 2 tablespoons honey
- 2 tablespoons warm water

Preparation:

1. Mix hoisin sauce with the rest of the marinade ingredients in a bowl.
2. Add star anise, peppercorns, 1 tablespoon wine, ginger, spring onion, and cinnamon to a saucepan.
3. Sir, in water and cook the mixture to a boil.
4. Place the duck in the water and blanch it for 2 minutes.
5. Drain and pat dry the duck, then leaves it in a colander to dry for 6 hours.
6. Place this duck in the Air Fryer basket and spray it with cooking oil.
7. Return the Air Fryer basket to the Air Fryer.

8. Select the Roast mode at 350 degrees F for 35 minutes.
9. Brush the duck with honey and cook for another 15 minutes.
10. Serve warm with hoisin sauce, scallion, and cucumber.

Serving Suggestion: Serve with warm corn tortilla and beetroot salad.

Variation Tip: Stuff duck with lemon or orange wedges.

Nutritional Information Per Serving:

Calories 223 | Fat 11.7g |Sodium 721mg | Carbs 13.6g | Fiber 0.7g | Sugar 8g | Protein 15.7g

11. Pickled Chicken Fillet

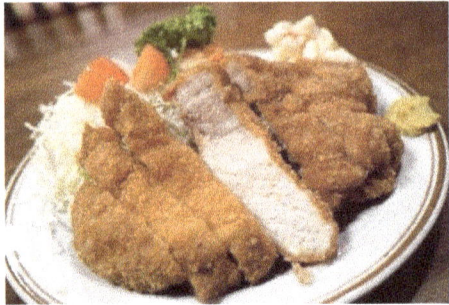

Prep Time: 15 minutes.
Cook Time: 20 minutes.
Serves: 2

Ingredients:

- 1-pound chicken fillets
- 1 cup pickle juice
- 1 cup flour
- 1 teaspoon garlic powder
- 1 teaspoon paprika
- 1 teaspoon basil
- 1 teaspoon salt
- 1 teaspoon pepper
- 1 tablespoon peanut oil
- 1/2 cup milk
- 1 egg

Preparation:

1. Soak the chicken fillets in the pickle juice for 1 hour.
2. Drain the chicken and keep it aside.
3. Mix dry ingredients in one bowl and beat egg with milk in another bowl.
4. Coat the chicken with flour mixture, then dip in the egg mixture.
5. Repeat the flour and egg coating to coat well.
6. Place the coated chicken fillets in the Air Fryer basket and spray with cooking oil.
7. Return the Air Fryer basket to the Air Fryer.
8. Select the Air Fry mode at 390 degrees F for 20 minutes.
9. Flip the chicken once cooked halfway through and resume cooking.
10. Serve warm.

Serving Suggestion: Serve with tomato ketchup or chili sauce.

Variation Tip: Use buttermilk instead of fresh milk.

Nutritional Information Per Serving:
Calories 456 | Fat 16.4g |Sodium 1321mg | Carbs 19.2g | Fiber 2.2g | Sugar 4.2g | Protein 55.2g

12. Savory Chicken Thighs

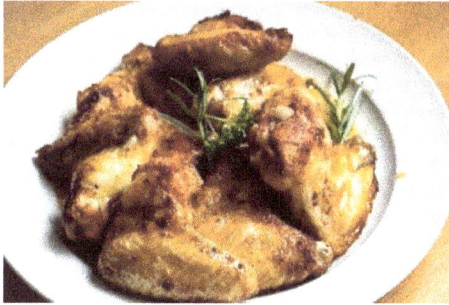

Prep Time: 15 minutes.
Cook Time: 25 minutes.
Serves: 6

Ingredients:

- 2 tablespoons garlic powder
- 2 tablespoons onion powder
- 2 tablespoons chili powder
- 1 tablespoon mustard powder
- 2 tablespoons kosher salt
- 1 tablespoon ground black pepper
- 4 cups buttermilk
- 2 bone-in chicken thighs
- 2 bone-in chicken breasts, cut in half
- 4 cups all-purpose flour
- 1/2 cup canola oil
- 2 tablespoons dark brown sugar
- 3 tablespoons paprika
- 2 teaspoons cayenne pepper

Preparation:

1. Mix onion, garlic, mustard powder, salt, black pepper, and chili in a bowl.
2. Whisk half of the spice mixture along with buttermilk to a plastic bag.
3. Place the chicken in this bag, seal, and shake well to coat.
4. Refrigerate the chicken for 8 hours or overnight.
5. Remove the chicken from the marinade and keep it aside.
6. Mix the remaining spice mixture with flour mixture in a shallow bowl.

7. Coat the chicken pieces lightly with the dry flour mixture and shake off the excess.
8. Place the coated chicken pieces in the Air Fryer basket and spray it with cooking oil.
9. Return the Air Fryer basket to the Air Fryer.
10. Select the Air Fry mode at 360 degrees F for 25 minutes.
11. Flip the chicken once cooked halfway through.
12. Meanwhile, mix ½ cup canola oil, cayenne pepper, paprika, and brown sugar in a bowl.
13. Pour this mixture over the cooked chicken and serve warm.

Serving Suggestion: Serve with tomato ketchup or chili sauce.

Variation Tip: Rub the chicken with garlic cloves before seasoning.

Nutritional Information Per Serving:

Calories 546 | Fat 33.1g |Sodium 1201mg | Carbs 30g | Fiber 2.4g | Sugar 9.7g | Protein 32g

13. Balsamic Chicken Thighs

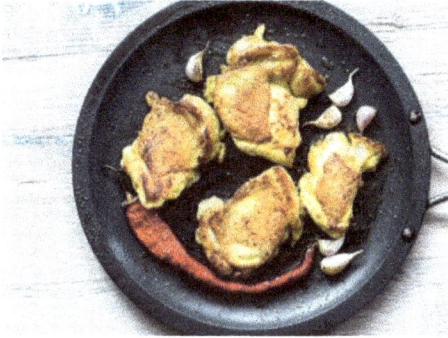

Prep Time: 15 minutes.
Cook Time: 14 minutes.
Serves: 4

Ingredients:

- 4 boneless skinless chicken thighs
- 1/4 cup lemon juice
- 1/4 cup coarse ground mustard
- 1/4 cup balsamic vinaigrette
- 1 teaspoon kosher salt
- 1 teaspoon dried rosemary leaves
- 1/2-1 teaspoon black pepper

Preparation:

1. Mix lemon juice, mustard, vinaigrette, salt, rosemary, and black pepper in a bowl.
2. Add chicken thighs and mix well to coat.
3. Cover and refrigerate for 2 hours for marination.
4. Set the seasoned chicken in the Air Fryer basket and spray with cooking oil.
5. Return the Air Fryer basket to the Air Fryer.
6. Select the Air Fry mode at 400 degrees F for 14 minutes.
7. Flip the chicken once cooked halfway through. And resume cooking.
8. Serve warm.

Serving Suggestion: Serve with cream cheese or onion dip.

Variation Tip: Rub the chicken with garlic cloves before seasoning.

Nutritional Information Per Serving:
Calories 331 | Fat 17g |Sodium 825mg | Carbs 1.7g | Fiber 0.3g | Sugar 1.3g | Protein 41g

14. Chicken Broccoli

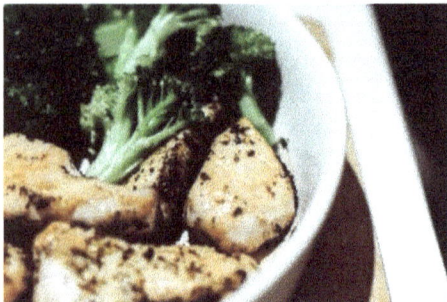

Prep Time: 15 minutes.
Cook Time: 20 minutes.
Serves: 4

Ingredients:

- ¼ pound broccoli, florets
- 1/2 medium onion, thick
- 2 tablespoons olive oil
- 1/2 teaspoon garlic powder
- 1 tablespoon ginger, minced
- 1 tablespoon soy sauce
- 1 teaspoon sesame seed oil
- 2 teaspoons rice vinegar
- 2 teaspoons hot sauce
- 1-pound boneless chicken breast, diced
- Salt, to taste
- Black pepper, to taste
- Lemon wedges

Preparation:

1. Mix olive oil, garlic powder, ginger, soy sauce, sesame oil, rice vinegar, hot sauce, salt, and black pepper in a large bowl.
2. Toss in chicken pieces, broccoli, and onion, then mix well to coat.
3. Spread the chicken and veggie mixture in the Air Fryer basket.
4. Return the Air Fryer basket to the Air Fryer.
5. Select the Air Fry mode at 380 degrees F for 20 minutes.
6. Toss the chicken once cooked halfway through.
7. Serve warm.

Serving Suggestion: Serve with warm tortilla and Greek salad.

Variation Tip: Add steamed edamame to the mixture.

Nutritional Information Per Serving:

Calories 310 | Fat 17g |Sodium 397mg | Carbs 4.7g | Fiber 1.3g | Sugar 1.3g | Protein 34.2g

15. Breaded Chicken Tenders

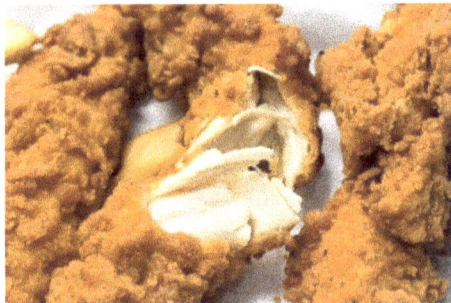

Prep Time: 10 minutes.

Cook Time: 20 minutes.

Serves: 6

Ingredients:

- 1 cup buttermilk
- 1/2 teaspoon hot sauce
- 2 pounds chicken tenders
- 1 cup all-purpose flour
- 1 ½ teaspoon Stone House Seasoning
- Cooking spray

Preparation:

1. Mix buttermilk with hot sauce in a large bowl.
2. Add chicken tenders, mix well and cover to refrigerate overnight.
3. Mix flour with stone house seasoning in a shallow bowl.
4. Stir in ¼ of the buttermilk marinade and mix well until smooth.
5. Dip the chicken tenders in the prepared batter to coat.
6. Place the coated chicken tenders in the Air Fryer basket and spray with cooking oil.
7. Return the Air Fryer basket to the Air Fryer.
8. Select the Air Fry mode at 370 degrees F for 20 minutes.
9. Flip the tenders once cooked halfway through, then resume cooking.
10. Serve warm.

Serving Suggestion: Serve with tomato ketchup or chili sauce.

Variation Tip: Use poultry seasoning for breading.

Nutritional Information Per Serving:

Calories 379 | Fat 12g |Sodium 184mg | Carbs 18g | Fiber 0.6g | Sugar 2g | Protein 47.2g

16. Ranch Chicken Wings

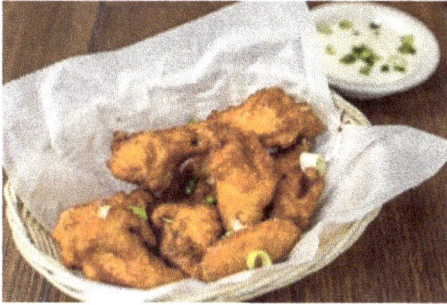

Prep Time: 15 minutes.

Cook Time: 20 minutes.

Serves: 4

Ingredients:

- 1 lb chicken wings
- 1 tablespoon Ranch seasoning mix
- 1 tablespoon garlic powder
- 2 tablespoon mayonnaise

Preparation:

1. Wash and pat dry 1 lb. chicken wings with a paper towel.
2. Mix mayonnaise with spices in a large bowl.
3. Stir in chicken wings and mix well to coat.
4. Cover and marinate the chicken for 15 minutes. in the refrigerator.
5. Place the chicken wings in the Air Fryer basket and spray them with cooking oil.
6. Return the Air Fryer basket to the Air Fryer.
7. Select the Air Fry mode at 400 degrees F for 20 minutes.
8. Flip the wings once cooked halfway through and resume cooking.
9. Serve warm.

Serving Suggestion: Serve with tomato ketchup or chili sauce.

Variation Tip: Use garlic mayonnaise.

Nutritional Information Per Serving:

Calories 251 | Fat 11g |Sodium 150mg | Carbs 3.3g | Fiber 0.2g | Sugar 1g | Protein 33.2g

Chapter 6: Beef, Pork, and Lamb

1. Air Fried Steaks

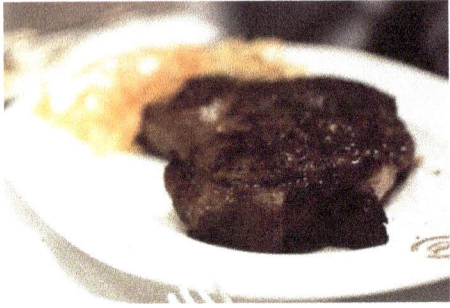

Prep Time: 10 minutes.

Cook Time: 15 minutes.

Serves: 2

Ingredients:

- 2 beef steaks
- 2 tablespoons avocado oil
- 1 tablespoon steak rub

Preparation:

1. Rub the steaks with oil and steam rub.
2. Place the steaks in the Air Fryer basket. And spray with cooking spray.
3. Return the Air Fryer basket to the Air Fryer.
4. Select the Air Fry mode at 400 degrees F for 15 minutes.
5. Flip the steaks once cooked halfway through and resume cooking.
6. Serve warm.

Serving Suggestion: Serve with sautéed leeks or cabbages.

Variation Tip: Rub the steaks with garlic cloves before seasoning.

Nutritional Information Per Serving:

Calories 400 | Fat 32g |Sodium 721mg | Carbs 2.6g | Fiber 0g | Sugar 0g | Protein 27.4g

2. Beef Fajitas

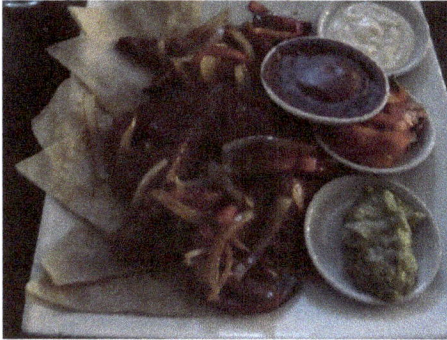

Prep Time: 10 minutes.
Cook Time: 10 minutes.
Serves: 4

Ingredients:

- 1-pound Angus beef skirt steak
- 1 red bell pepper, diced
- 1 green bell pepper, diced
- 1 yellow bell pepper, diced
- 1 orange bell pepper, diced
- 1/4 cup sweet onion, diced
- 4 tablespoons fajita seasoning
- Corn tortillas

Preparation:

1. Slice the steaks against the grain.
2. Toss the beef and veggies with fajita seasoning in a large bowl.
3. Spread the beef mixture in the Air Fryer basket and spray with cooking oil.
4. Return the Air Fryer basket to the Air Fryer.
5. Select the Air Fry mode at 390 degrees F for 10 minutes.
6. Toss the fajita once cooked halfway through and resume cooking.
7. Serve warm in a warm tortilla.

Serving Suggestion: Serve with avocado dip.

Variation Tip: Add sliced carrots and zucchini to the fajitas as well.

Nutritional Information Per Serving:

Calories 316 | Fat 12.2g |Sodium 587mg | Carbs 12.2g | Fiber 1g | Sugar 1.8g | Protein 25.8g

3. Tarragon Lamb Chops

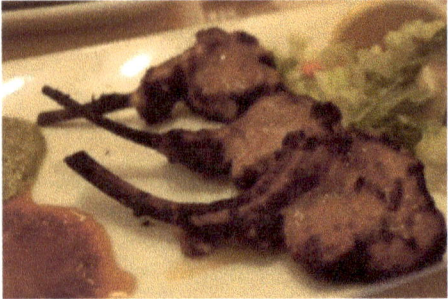

Prep Time: 15 minutes.

Cook Time: 15 minutes.

Serves: 8

Ingredients:

- 8 lamb loin chops, 1 ¼" wide
- 2 tablespoons mustard
- ½ teaspoon olive oil
- 1 teaspoon dried tarragon
- 1 tablespoon lemon juice
- Salt and black pepper

Preparation:

1. At 390 degrees F, preheat your Ninja Air Fryer on Air Fry mode.
2. Mix mustard, tarragon, olive oil, and lemon juice in a small bowl.
3. Wash and pat dry the lamb chops and rub them with mustard mixture.
4. Place the chops in the Air Fryer basket and spray them with cooking oil.
5. Return the Air Fryer basket to the Air Fryer and cook for 15 minutes.
6. Flip the chops once cooked halfway through and resume cooking.
7. Serve warm.

Serving Suggestion: Serve with tomato ketchup or chili sauce.

Variation Tip: Rub the lamb with garlic cloves before seasoning.

Nutritional Information Per Serving:

Calories 336 | Fat 27.1g |Sodium 66mg | Carbs 1.1g | Fiber 0.4g | Sugar 0.2g | Protein 19.7g

4. Herbed Lamb Chops

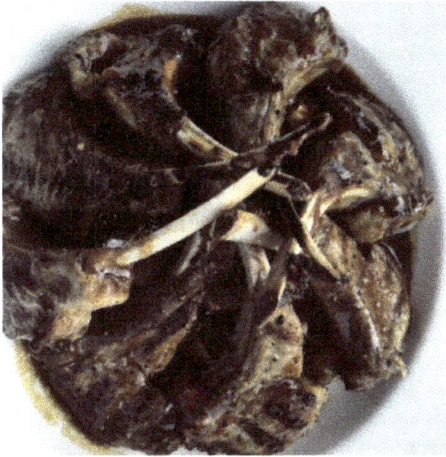

Prep Time: 15 minutes.

Cook Time: 9 minutes.

Serves: 2

Ingredients:

- 1 teaspoon rosemary
- 1 teaspoon thyme
- 1 teaspoon oregano
- 1 teaspoon salt
- 1 teaspoon coriander
- 2 tablespoons olive oil
- 2 tablespoons lemon juice
- 1-pound lamb chops

Preparation:

1. Mix rosemary, thyme, oregano, salt, coriander, lemon juice, and olive oil in a bowl.
2. Rub this mixture well over the chops liberally.
3. Place the chops in the Air Fryer basket and spray them with cooking oil.
4. Return the Air Fryer basket to the Air Fryer.
5. Select the Air Fry mode at 390 degrees F for 9 minutes.
6. Flip the chops once cooked halfway through and resume cooking.
7. Serve warm.

Serving Suggestion: Serve with fresh vegetable salad.

Variation Tip: Rub the lamb chops with garlic cloves before seasoning.

Nutritional Information Per Serving:

Calories 551 | Fat 31g |Sodium 1329mg | Carbs 1.5g | Fiber 0.8g | Sugar 0.4g | Protein 64g

5. Roasted Lamb Rack

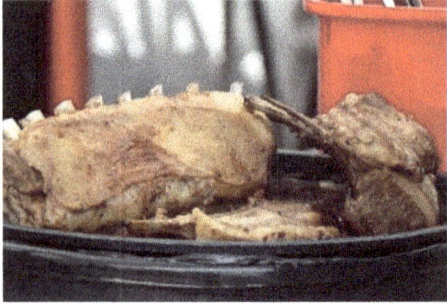

Prep Time: 15 minutes.

Cook Time: 50 minutes.

Serves: 4

Ingredients:

- 1 2/3 pounds rack of lamb
- Salt and black pepper, to taste
- ¼ pound dry breadcrumbs
- 1 teaspoon garlic, grated
- 1/2 teaspoon salt
- 1 teaspoon cumin seeds
- 1 teaspoon ground cumin
- 1 teaspoon oil
- Grated lemon rind
- 1 egg, beaten

Preparation:

1. At 400 degrees F, preheat your Ninja Air Fryer on Air Fry mode.
2. Rub the lamb rack with black pepper and salt, then keep it aside.
3. Mix breadcrumbs with ½ teaspoons salt, ground cumin, cumin seeds, lemon rind, oil, and grated garlic in a bowl.
4. Beat egg in one bowl and keep it aside.
5. Dip the lamb rack in the egg and coat with the breadcrumb's mixture.
6. Place the coated lamb in the Air Fryer basket.
7. Return the Air Fryer basket to the Air Fryer.
8. Select the Air Fry mode at 400 degrees F for 50 minutes.
9. Flip the lamb once cooked halfway through.
10. Serve warm.

Serving Suggestion: Serve with warm corn tortilla and crouton salad.

Variation Tip: Rub the lamb rack with garlic cloves before seasoning.

Nutritional Information Per Serving:

Calories 410 | Fat 17.8g |Sodium 619mg | Carbs 21g | Fiber 1.4g | Sugar 1.8g | Protein 38.4g

6. Crusted Pork Chops

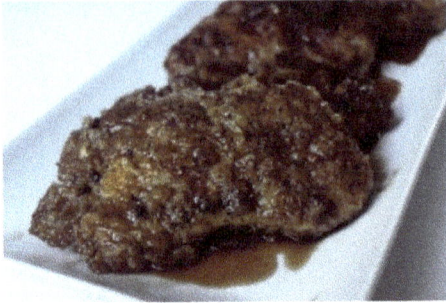

Prep Time: 10 minutes.

Cook Time: 14 minutes.

Serves: 3

Ingredients:

- 1 lb boneless pork chops
- 3 tablespoons olive oil
- 1 tablespoon Cajun seasoning
- ¼ cup parmesan, grated
- ½ teaspoon of sea salt

Preparation:

1. Pat dry boneless pork chops with a paper towel.
2. Mix parmesan, seasonings, and salt in a shallow bowl.
3. Rub the prepared pork chops with olive oil and the parmesan mixture.
4. Place the chops in the Air Fryer basket and spray them with cooking oil.
5. Return the Air Fryer basket to the Air Fryer.
6. Select the Air Fry mode at 375 degrees F for 14 minutes.
7. Flip the chops once cooked halfway through and resume cooking.
8. Serve warm.

Serving Suggestion: Serve boiled rice or steamed cauliflower rice.

Variation Tip: Rub the chops with garlic cloves before seasoning.

Nutritional Information Per Serving:

Calories 396 | Fat 23.2g |Sodium 622mg | Carbs 0.7g | Fiber 0g | Sugar 0g | Protein 45.6g

7. Bacon-Wrapped Pork Chop

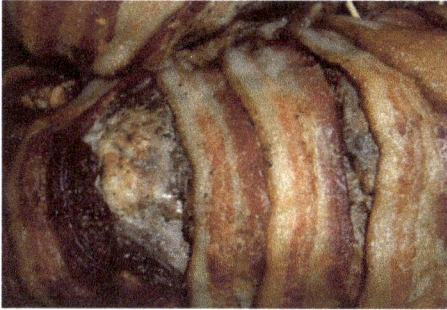

Prep Time: 15 minutes.
Cook Time: 10 minutes.
Serves: 4

Ingredients:

- 4 pork chops
- 8 bacon strips
- ½ cup brown sugar
- 1 tablespoon salt
- 1 tablespoon garlic salt
- ½ tablespoon chili powder
- ½ tablespoon paprika

Preparation:

1. At 400 degrees F, preheat your Ninja Air Fryer on Air Fry mode.
2. Mix brown sugar, salt, garlic salt, chili powder, and paprika in a bowl.
3. Rub the chops with half of this mixture.
4. Wrap each chop with two bacon strips and seal with a toothpick.
5. Place the chops in the Air Fryer basket.
6. Return the Air Fryer basket to the Air Fryer and cook for 10 minutes.
7. Flip the chops once cooked halfway through and resume cooking.
8. Serve warm.

Serving Suggestion: Serve with tomato ketchup or chili sauce.

Variation Tip: Rub the chops with garlic cloves before seasoning.

Nutritional Information Per Serving:
Calories 437 | Fat 28g |Sodium 1221mg | Carbs 22.3g | Fiber 0.9g | Sugar 8g | Protein 30.3g

8. Ranch Pork Tenderloin

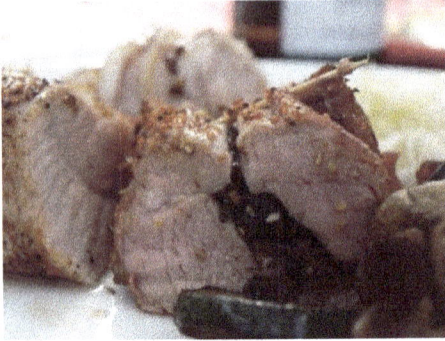

Prep Time: 10 minutes.
Cook Time: 20 minutes.
Serves: 2

Ingredients:

- 1-pound pork tenderloin
- 2 tablespoons ranch seasoning
- 1 teaspoon salt
- 2 teaspoons avocado oil

Homemade ranch seasoning

- ¼ cup parsley dried
- 1 teaspoon dill dried
- 2 teaspoons garlic powder
- 2 teaspoons onion, minced
- 1 tablespoon chives, dried
- 1 teaspoon mustard powder
- 1 teaspoon black pepper

Preparation:

1. Mix parsley, dill, garlic powder, minced onion, dried chives, mustard powder, and black pepper in a bowl to prepare the ranch seasoning.
2. Rub the pork with avocado oil, sea salt, and ranch seasoning.
3. Place the pork tenderloin in the Air Fryer basket.
4. Return the Air Fryer basket to the Air Fryer.
5. Select the Air Fry mode at 400 degrees F for 20 minutes.
6. Flip the pork once cooked halfway through and resume cooking.
7. Serve warm.

Serving Suggestion: Serve with sautéed zucchini and green beans.

Variation Tip: Rub the pork with garlic cloves before seasoning.

Nutritional Information Per Serving:

Calories 352 | Fat 9.1g |Sodium 1294mg | Carbs 3.9g | Fiber 1g | Sugar 1g | Protein 61g

9. Air Fried Pork Belly

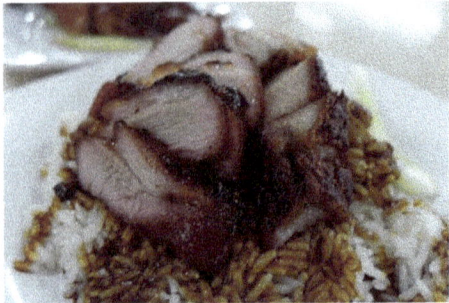

Prep Time: 10 minutes.

Cook Time: 15 minutes.

Serves: 6

Ingredients:

- 12 pork belly slices
- 1 cup BBQ sauce

Preparation:

1. Toss pork bell strips with BBQ sauce in a bowl.
2. Spread the pork belly slices in the Air Fryer basket.
3. Return the Air Fryer basket to the Air Fryer.
4. Select the Air Fry mode at 400 degrees F for 15 minutes.
5. Flip the pork strips once cooked halfway through and resume cooking.
6. Serve warm.

Serving Suggestion: Serve on top of boiled white rice.

Variation Tip: Add Worcestershire sauce and honey to taste.

Nutritional Information Per Serving:

Calories 374 | Fat 25g |Sodium 275mg | Carbs 7.3g | Fiber 0g | Sugar 6g | Protein 12.3g

10. Beef Kabobs

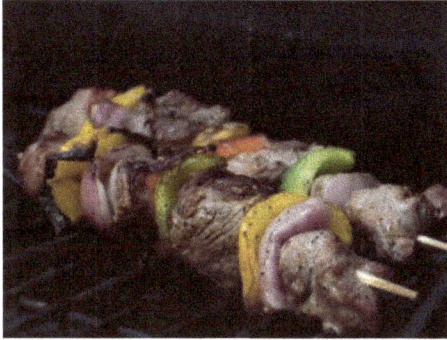

Prep Time: 15 minutes.
Cook Time: 10 minutes.
Serves: 6

Ingredients:

- 1 ½ pound sirloin steak, diced
- 1 large bell pepper, cut into squares
- 1 large red onion, cut into squares

Marinade:

- 4 tablespoons olive oil
- 2 garlic cloves, minced
- 1 tablespoon lemon juice
- 1/2 teaspoon salt
- 1/2 teaspoon black pepper

Preparation:

1. Mix olive oil, garlic, lemon juice, black pepper, and salt in a bowl.
2. Toss in sirloin, bell pepper, and red onion, then mix well.
3. Thread the beef, bell pepper, and onion alternately on the wooden skewers.
4. Place the skewers in the Air Fryer basket.
5. Return the Air Fryer basket to the Air Fryer.
6. Select the Air Fry mode at 400 degrees F for 10 minutes.
7. Flip the skewers once cooked halfway through and resume cooking.
8. Serve warm.

Serving Suggestion: Serve with tomato ketchup or chili sauce.

Variation Tip: Add diced zucchini and cherry tomatoes to the skewers as well.

Nutritional Information Per Serving:
Calories 310 | Fat 17g |Sodium 271mg | Carbs 4.3g | Fiber 0.9g | Sugar 2.1g | Protein 35g

11. Herb Crusted Beef Roast

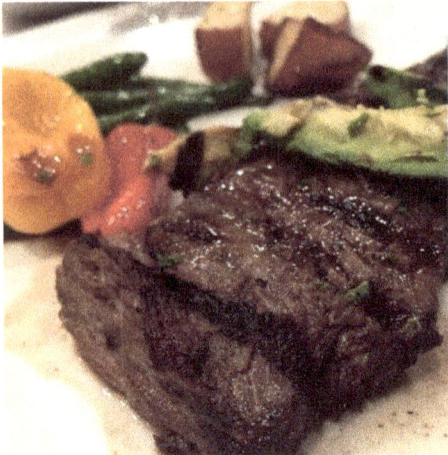

Prep Time: 15 minutes.
Cook Time: 75 minutes.
Serves: 4

Ingredients:

- 2-pound beef roast
- 2 teaspoons garlic powder
- 2 teaspoons onion salt
- 2 teaspoons parsley
- 2 teaspoons thyme
- 2 teaspoons basil
- ½ tablespoon salt
- 1 teaspoon black pepper
- 1 tablespoon olive oil

Preparation:

1. At 390 degrees F, preheat your Ninja Air Fryer on Air Fry mode.
2. Mix onion salt, garlic powder, basil, salt, black pepper, thyme, and parsley in a bowl.
3. Rub olive oil and spice mixture over the beef roast.
4. Place the beef in the Air Fryer basket.
5. Return the Air Fryer basket to the Air Fryer.
6. Select the Air Fry mode at 360 degrees F for 15 minutes.
7. Flip the roast and continue cooking for another 60 minutes.
8. Slice and serve warm.

Serving Suggestion: Serve with sautéed green beans and cherry tomatoes.

Variation Tip: Rub the roast with garlic cloves before seasoning.

Nutritional Information Per Serving:

Calories 459 | Fat 17.7g |Sodium 1516mg | Carbs 1.7g | Fiber 0.5g | Sugar 0.4g | Protein 69.2g

12. Herbed Ribeye

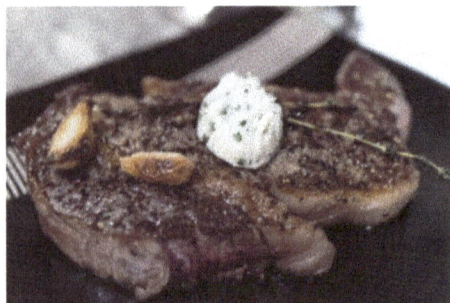

Prep Time: 10 minutes.
Cook Time: 14 minutes.
Serves: 4

Ingredients:

- 4 tablespoons butter, softened
- 2 garlic cloves, minced
- 2 teaspoons parsley, chopped
- 1 teaspoon chives, chopped
- 1 teaspoon thyme, chopped
- 1 teaspoon rosemary, chopped
- 1 (2 lbs.) bone-in ribeye
- Kosher salt, to taste
- Freshly ground black pepper, to taste

Preparation:

1. Mix softened butter with parsley, chives, thyme, rosemary, and garlic in a plastic bag.
2. Rub the ribeye with salt, and black pepper, then place them in the plastic bag.
3. Seal the bag and shake well to coat.
4. Refrigerate the ribeye for 20 minutes. for marination.
5. Place the ribeye in the Air Fryer basket.
6. Return the Air Fryer basket to the Air Fryer.
7. Select the Air Fry mode at 400 degrees F for 14 minutes.
8. Flip the ribeye once cooked halfway through and resume cooking.
9. Serve warm and enjoy.

Serving Suggestion: Serve the ribeye with a dollop of cream cheese dip on top.

Variation Tip: Rub the steak with garlic cloves before seasoning.

Nutritional Information Per Serving:
Calories 264 | Fat 17g |Sodium 129mg | Carbs 0.9g | Fiber 0.3g | Sugar 0g | Protein 27g

Chapter 7: Dessert Recipes

1. Hand Pies

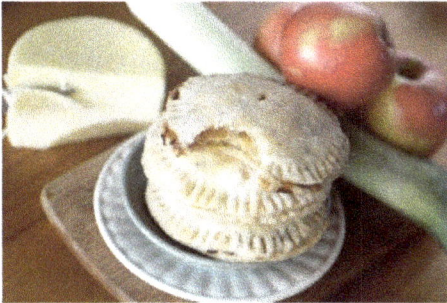

Prep Time: 20 minutes.
Cook Time: 14 minutes.
Serves: 8

Ingredients:

- ¼ cup blueberry jam
- ¼ cup fresh blueberries
- 1 lemon, zest
- Flour for dusting
- 2 pie crusts, softened
- 1 egg
- 2 tablespoons sugar
- ¼ teaspoons ground cinnamon
- Oil for spritzing
- ¼ cup powdered sugar

Preparation:

1. Mix blueberries with lemon zest and jam in a medium bowl.
2. Spread each pie dough on a floured surface and cut 8 circles using a 3 inches cookie cutter.
3. Add 1 tablespoon of blueberry mixture at the center of the eight circles.
4. Place the remaining circles on top and crimp their edges with a fork to seal.
5. Brush the pies with egg and drizzle cinnamon and sugar on top.
6. Place the pies in the Air Fryer basket, use a fry rack to adjust the pies.
7. Return the Air Fryer basket to the Air Fryer.
8. Select the Air Fry mode at 360 degrees F for 14 minutes.
9. Flip the pies once cooked halfway through and resume cooking.
10. Serve warm.

Serving Suggestion: Serve with apple sauce.

Variation Tip: Add shredded apples to the filling.

Nutritional Information Per Serving:

Calories 284 | Fat 16g |Sodium 252mg | Carbs 31.6g | Fiber 0.9g | Sugar 6.6g | Protein 3.7g

2. Cheesecake Chimichangas

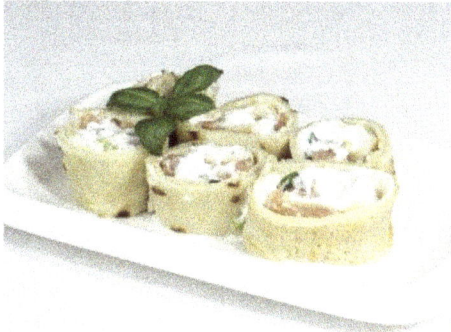

Prep Time: 15 minutes.
Cook Time: 8 minutes.
Serves: 6

Ingredients:

- 1/4 cup sour cream
- 1 ½ tablespoon granulated sugar
- 1 teaspoon vanilla extract
- 8 strawberries, quartered
- 1 banana, peeled and sliced
- 8 flour tortillas
- 8 teaspoons Nutella
- Olive oil spray
- 1 (8 ounces) cream cheese brick, softened
- 3 tablespoons butter, melted

Cinnamon sugar:

- 2 tablespoons sugar
- 2 tablespoons cinnamon ground

Preparation:

1. Beat cream cheese, sour cream, vanilla, sugar, strawberries, and banana in a bowl.
2. Spread the tortillas on the working surface.
3. Divide the cream mixture onto the tortillas and divide Nutella on top.
4. Roll the tortillas like a burrito and place it in the Air Fryer basket.
5. Return the Air Fryer basket to the Air Fryer.
6. Select the Air Fry mode at 360 degrees F for 8 minutes.
7. Slice the rolls into 1-inch thick pieces and place them on the plate.
8. Drizzle melted butter and cinnamon sugar on top.
9. Serve.

Serving Suggestion: Serve with strawberry jam.

Variation Tip: Add mashed blueberries to the filling.

Nutritional Information Per Serving:

Calories 391 | Fat 24g |Sodium 142mg | Carbs 38.5g | Fiber 3.5g | Sugar 21g | Protein 6.6g

3. Baked Cinnamon Apples

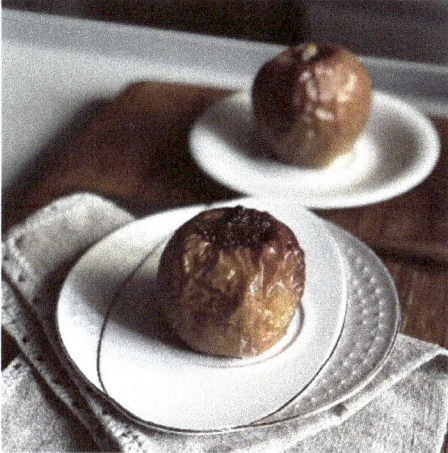

Prep Time: 10 minutes.
Cook Time: 20 minutes.
Serves: 4

Ingredients:

- 4 apples
- 2 teaspoons honey
- 6 teaspoons raisins
- 2 teaspoons walnuts, chopped
- ½ teaspoons cinnamon

Preparation:

1. Place apples in a six inches baking pan.
2. Drizzle honey, raisins, walnuts, and cinnamon on top.
3. Place the pan in the Air Fryer basket.
4. Return the Air Fryer basket to the Air Fryer.
5. Select the Air Fry mode at 350 degrees F for 20 minutes.
6. Serve.

Serving Suggestion: Serve with a dollop of vanilla ice-cream.

Variation Tip: Stuff chopped nuts in the apple core.

Nutritional Information Per Serving:
Calories 149 | Fat 1.2g | Sodium 3mg | Carbs 37.6g | Fiber 5.8g | Sugar 29g | Protein 1.1g

4. Apple Fritters

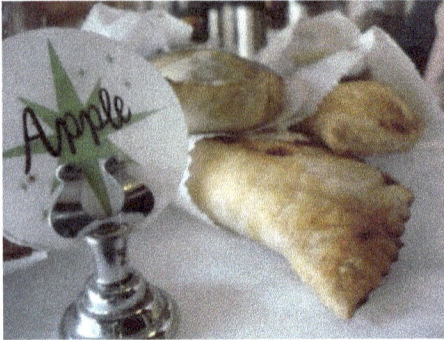

Prep Time: 15 minutes.
Cook Time: 8 minutes.
Serves: 6

Ingredients:

- ½ cup of sugar
- ½ teaspoon ground cinnamon
- 1 cup apple, peeled and chopped
- 1 can (10 oz) Pillsbury refrigerated biscuits (5 biscuits)
- 3 tablespoons butter, melted

Preparation:

1. Cut 2- eight inches rounds out of a parchment paper.
2. Spread one 8 inches round in the Air Fryer basket and grease it with cooking spray.
3. Mix cinnamon ground with sugar in a small bowl.
4. Toss in chopped apple, then mix well.
5. Make 5 biscuits out of the dough and cut each biscuit into 2 layers.
6. Spread each round into 4 inches rounds.
7. Add 1 tablespoon apple mixture at the center of each round.
8. Fold the edges of each round over the filling and pinch to seal.
9. Brush the refrigerated biscuits with melted butter and place them in the Air Fryer basket in batches.
10. Place the other parchment paper round on top and return the Air Fryer basket to the Air Fryer.
11. Select the Air Fry mode at 325 degrees F for 8 minutes.
12. Flip the biscuits once cooked halfway through.
13. Drizzle butter and cinnamon sugar on top.
14. Serve.

Serving Suggestion: Serve with a dollop of sweet cream dip

Variation Tip: Add chopped raisins and nuts to the filling.

Nutritional Information Per Serving:

Calories 327 | Fat 14.2g |Sodium 672mg | Carbs 47.2g | Fiber 1.7g | Sugar 24.8g | Protein 4.4g

5. Air Fried Brownies

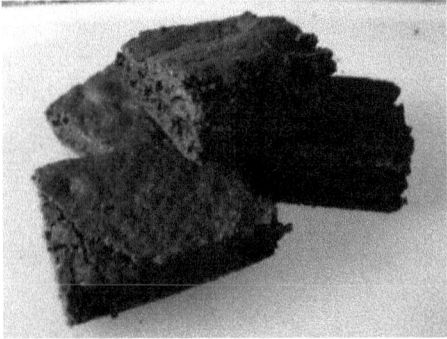

Prep Time: 15 minutes.
Cook Time: 15 minutes.
Serves: 8

Ingredients:

- ½ cup all-purpose flour
- 6 tablespoons cocoa powder
- ¾ cup of sugar
- ¼ cup butter, melted
- 2 large eggs
- 1 tablespoon vegetable oil
- ½ teaspoons vanilla extract
- ¼ teaspoons salt
- ¼ teaspoons baking powder

Preparation:

1. Grease a 7 inches baking pan with butter.
2. At 330 degrees F, preheat your Ninja Air Fryer on Air Fry mode.
3. Whisk vegetable oil, vanilla extract, and butter in a mixing bowl.
4. Stir in cocoa powder, sugar, eggs, vanilla, flour, salt, and baking powder.
5. Mix well until smooth, then pour into the baking pan.
6. Place this pan Air Fryer basket.
7. Return the Air Fryer basket to the Air Fryer.
8. Select the Air Fry mode at 330 degrees F for 15 minutes.
9. Slice and serve.

Serving Suggestion: Serve the hot brownie with a scoop of vanilla ice-cream.

Variation Tip: Add chopped nuts for a different texture.

Nutritional Information Per Serving:
Calories 192 | Fat 9.3g |Sodium 133mg | Carbs 27.1g | Fiber 1.4g | Sugar 19g | Protein 3.2g

6. Air Fried Churros

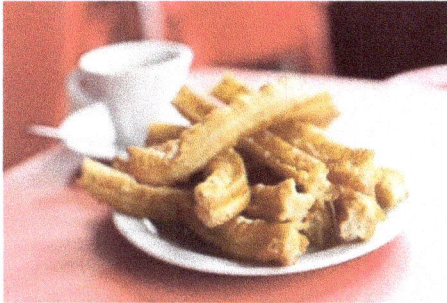

Prep Time: 20 minutes.
Cook Time: 12 minutes.
Serves:8

Ingredients:

- 1 cup of water
- 1/3 cup butter, cut into cubes
- 2 tablespoons granulated sugar
- 1/4 teaspoon salt
- 1 cup all-purpose flour
- 2 large eggs
- 1 teaspoon vanilla extract
- Oil spray

Cinnamon-sugar coating:

- 1/2 cup granulated sugar
- 3/4 teaspoons ground cinnamon

Preparation:

1. Boil water with sugar, salt, and butter in a saucepan over medium-high heat.
2. Reduce heat and add flour, then mix continuously until smooth.
3. Beat eggs with vanilla and add to the cooled flour batter.
4. Mix well with a hand mixer until it makes a thick batter.
5. Transfer the mixture to a piping bag.
6. Pipe the mixture on a baking sheet lined with parchment paper into 4 inches long churros.
7. Refrigerate the churros for 1 hour.
8. Place the churros in the Air Fryer basket and spray them with cooking oil.
9. Return the Air Fryer basket to the Air Fryer.
10. Select the Air Fry mode at 375 degrees F for 12 minutes.
11. Drizzle sugar and cinnamon on top.
12. Serve.

Serving Suggestion: Serve with chocolate syrup on the side.

Variation Tip: Add 1 teaspoon of cocoa powder to the churro batter before.

Nutritional Information Per Serving:

Calories 204 | Fat 9g |Sodium 91mg | Carbs 27g | Fiber 2.4g | Sugar 15g | Protein 1.3g

7. Funnel Cakes

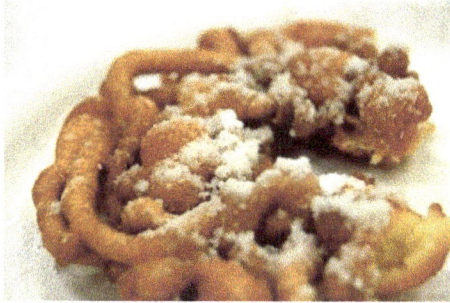

Prep Time: 20 minutes.
Cook Time: 4 minutes.
Serves: 4

Ingredients:

- 1 cup all-purpose flour
- 1 ¼ teaspoons baking powder
- 1/4 teaspoon salt
- 1/2 teaspoon ground cinnamon
- 1 cup Greek yogurt
- 1 teaspoon vanilla extract
- Vegetable oil spray
- Powdered sugar

Preparation:

1. Mix ¾ cup flour, salt, cinnamon, and baking powder in a bowl.
2. Add vanilla and yogurt, then mix well until it makes a smooth ball.
3. Transfer the prepared dough on a floured surface and roll the dough into a 1/4-inch-thick sheet.
4. Slice the sheet into 1-inch thick strips and use these strips to make funnel cakes.
5. Place the funnel cakes in the Air Fryer basket and spray with cooking oil.
6. Return the Air Fryer basket to the Air Fryer.
7. Select the Air Fry mode at 375 degrees F for 4 minutes.
8. Flip the cakes once cooked halfway through and resume cooking.
9. Serve with powdered sugar on top.

Serving Suggestion: Serve with chocolate syrup on the side.

Variation Tip: Add 2 teaspoons of cocoa powder to the batter.

Nutritional Information Per Serving:
Calories 157 | Fat 1.3g |Sodium 27mg | Carbs 1.3g | Fiber 1g | Sugar 2.2g | Protein 8.2g

8. Chocolate Chip Cookies

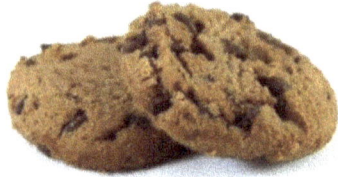

Prep Time: 15 minutes.

Cook Time: 15 minutes.

Serves: 12

Ingredients:

- 9 oz. self-rising flour
- 1 ½ oz. coconut sugar
- 3 oz. brown sugar
- 5 oz. butter
- 4 tablespoons honey
- 3 tablespoons milk
- 1 tablespoon cocoa powder
- 1 teaspoon vanilla essence
- 3 ½ oz. chocolate chips

Preparation:

1. At 360 degrees F, preheat your Ninja Air Fryer on Air Fry mode.
2. Beat sugars with butter in a mixing bowl using a hand mixer.
3. Stir in milk, vanilla, cocoa powder, honey, and flour.
4. Mix well and stir in chocolate chips.
5. Knead the cookie dough and divide it into 12 small cookies.
6. Place the cookies in the Air Fryer basket, in batches.
7. Return the Air Fryer basket to the Air Fryer.
8. Select the Air Fry mode at 360 degrees F for 15 minutes.
9. Allow the cookies to cool, then serve.

Serving Suggestion: Serve with a warming cup of hot chocolate.

Variation Tip: Use maple syrup instead of honey

Nutritional Information Per Serving:

Calories 258 | Fat 12.4g |Sodium 79mg | Carbs 34.3g | Fiber 1g | Sugar 17g | Protein 3.2g

9. Cinnamon Rolls

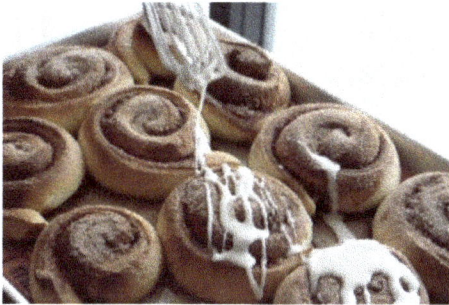

Prep Time: 15 minutes.
Cook Time: 7 minutes.
Serves: 6

Ingredients:

Cinnamon rolls:

- 1 tablespoon ground cinnamon
- ¾ stick unsalted butter softened
- 6 tablespoons brown sugar
- 1 sheet puff pastry, thawed

Icing:

- ½ cup powdered sugar
- 1 tablespoon milk
- 2 teaspoons lemon juice

Preparation:

1. Mix softened butter, sugar, and cinnamon in a small bowl.
2. At 400 degrees F, preheat your Ninja Air Fryer on Air Fry mode.
3. Roll the pastry dough on a working surface.
4. Brush the top with butter and drizzle brown sugar and cinnamon on top.
5. Roll the pastry and cut the log into a 1-inch thick piece.
6. Place the prepared cinnamon rolls in the Air Fryer basket.
7. Return the Air Fryer basket to the Air Fryer.
8. Select the Air Fry mode at 400 degrees F for 7 minutes.
9. Flip the cinnamon rolls once cooked halfway through.
10. Mix sugar with milk and lemon juice in a bowl.
11. Pour this mixture over the cinnamon rolls.
12. Serve.

Serving Suggestion: Serve a cup of spice latte or hot chocolate.

Variation Tip: Use brown swerve instead of sugar to reduce the carbs.

Nutritional Information Per Serving:

Calories 175 | Fat 13.1g |Sodium 154mg | Carbs 14g | Fiber 0.8g | Sugar 8.9g | Protein 0.7g

Conclusion

Are you ready to take these recipes to the next level? It's about time that you give these recipes a try and surprise your family and loved ones with the ultimate crispy delights. Air Frying is the need of today; we can't really rely on the old deep-frying methods when it comes to keeping good health. High blood cholesterol and cardiac disease are some of the most rampant health issues in today's age because of our busy lifestyle and oily food make it difficult to keep the blood cholesterol maintained. But frying was never really possible before until the new Air Frying technology swooped in and took the world by a storm. Now Air Fryers has become the need for every household. And ever since the Air Fryers were converted into these small and compact multipurpose cooking appliances, they became more relevant than ever. Today, you can cook all sorts of meal in these Air Fryers without the fear of overcooking, burning or undercooking your food because these Air Fryers comes with a digitally controlled heating mechanism which blows hot air through the food at a set temperature for a set cooking time.

Ninja Foodi, due to its effective heating technology and amazing designs, has been giving major competition to all its Air Fryer competitors in the market. Though there are several new models out in the market, nothing can beat the performance of the classic AF 101, which is super simple and easy to use, and yet it gives great results. From its cooking capacity to crisp technology, the Air Fryer has every feature to surprise the users.

So, if you were new to this whole idea of Air Frying or had been thinking of giving the Ninja Foodi Air Fryer a try, then this cookbook has provided a perfect compilation of the recipes that you can use every day or on special occasions. Each recipe is designed with easy to get basic ingredients and simple to follow instructions so that you will have a comfortable and memorable experience using your Ninja Food Air Fryer. These unique recipes will also help the Ninja foodi users keep their menu diverse and rich in flavors and aroma.